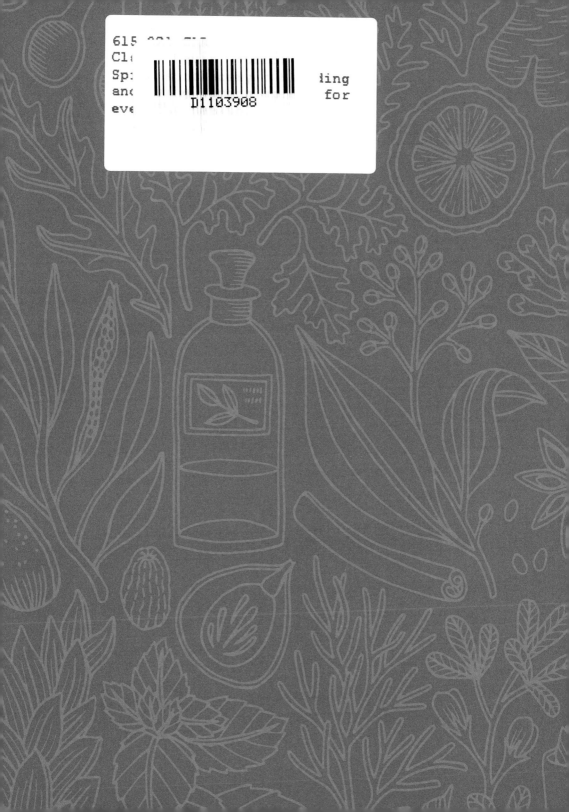

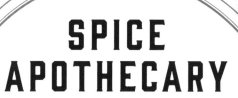

SPICE
APOTHECARY

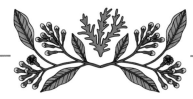

BLENDING AND USING
COMMON SPICES FOR
EVERYDAY HEALTH

BEVIN CLARE

Storey Publishing

The mission of Storey Publishing is to serve our customers by publishing practical information that encourages personal independence in harmony with the environment.

Edited by Carleen Madigan and Liz Bevilacqua
Art direction by Ash Austin
Book design by Kimberly Glyder
Text production by Jennifer Jepson Smith
Indexed by Samantha Miller

Cover photography by © Michael Piazza Photography/SAINT LUCY Represents, except for back (dished spices) by Mars Vilaubi
Interior photography by © Michael Piazza Photography/SAINT LUCY Represents
Additional photography by © Bevin Clare, 78 & 79; Courtesy of Funke Koleosho, 42; © margo555/stock.adobe.com, 97 left; Mars Vilaubi, 6, 87, 89 top, 90 right, 91, 94 right, 96 left, 97 right, 99 bottom left, 101 left; © MaxyM/Shutterstock.com, decorative labels, 10 and throughout; Courtesy of Michael Tims, 28; Courtesy of Patricia Howell, 142; © Sandeep Agarwal, 150
Photo styling by Ann Lewis
Food styling by Ash Austin
Cover and interior illustrations, including backgrounds, by © Andie Hanna
Diagram page 29 by Ash Austin

Storey books are available at special discounts when purchased in bulk for premiums and sales promotions as well as for fund-raising or educational use. Special editions or book excerpts can also be created to specification. For details, please call 800-827-8673, or send an email to sales@storey.com.

Storey Publishing
210 MASS MoCA Way
North Adams, MA 01247
storey.com

Printed in China through World Print
10 9 8 7 6 5 4 3 2 1

LIBRARY OF CONGRESS CATALOGING-IN-PUBLICATION DATA

Names: Clare, Bevin, author.
Title: Spice apothecary / Bevin Clare.
Description: North Adams : Storey Publishing, 2020. | Includes bibliographical references and index. | Summary: "Author Bevin Clare combines her training in herbalism and nutrition to guide readers in a return to the kitchen spice cabinet for better health and healing"—Provided by publisher.
Identifiers: LCCN 2019056609 (print) | LCCN 2019056610 (ebook) | ISBN 9781635860832 (paperback) | ISBN 9781635860887 (hardcover) | ISBN 9781635860849 (ebook)
Subjects: LCSH: Spices—Therapeutic use. | Spices—Health aspects. | Cooking (Herbs)
Classification: LCC RM666.H33 C623 2020 (print) | LCC RM666.H33 (ebook) | DDC 615.3/21—dc23
LC record available at https://lccn.loc.gov/2019056609
LC ebook record available at https://lccn.loc.gov/2019056610

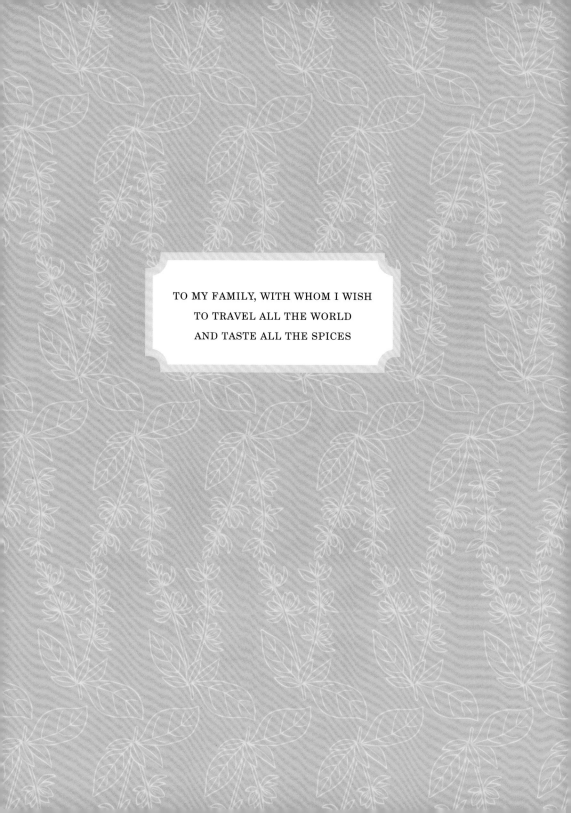

TO MY FAMILY, WITH WHOM I WISH
TO TRAVEL ALL THE WORLD
AND TASTE ALL THE SPICES

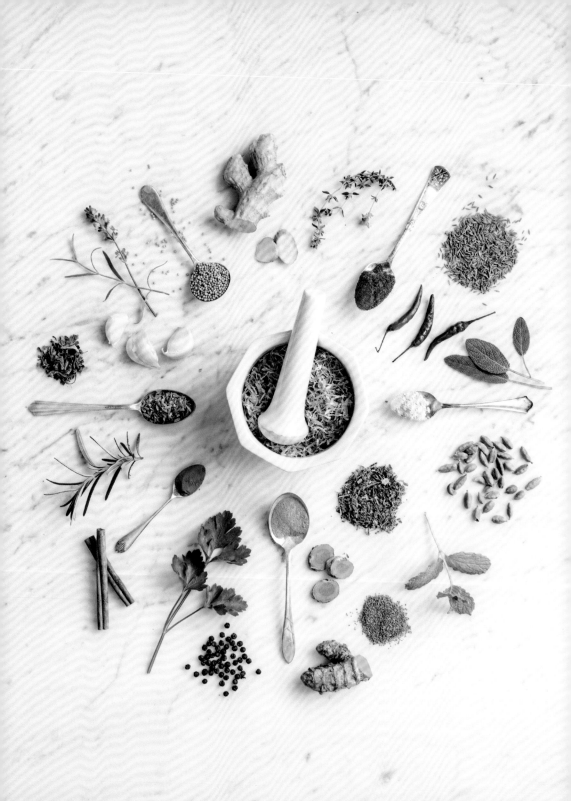

CONTENTS

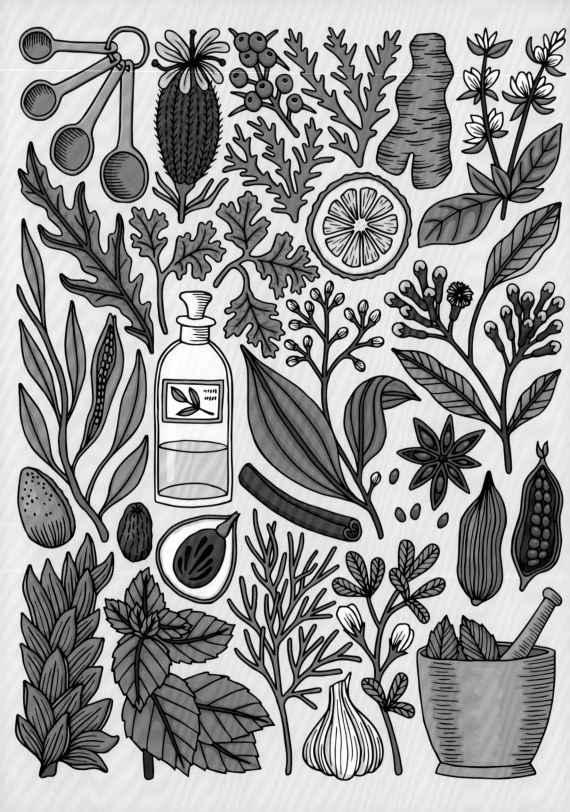

I HAVE BEEN ASKED HUNDREDS OF TIMES, "What do you take every day to stay healthy?" I imagine people have visions of me with cauldrons of bubbling medicines, or bowls of rainbow-colored capsules, or dozens of amber tincture bottles lined up on my kitchen table. When I tell people that the only medicines I take every day are things like garlic, cinnamon, black pepper, and basil, I can sometimes see a hint of disappointment. Just simple spices, when they thought they might discover the secret to youth or immortality.

But this is an underestimation of the power of culinary herbs and spices. How could something that tastes good be used medicinally? Could something that our grand-mothers and grandfathers cooked with every day be fundamental to good health?

What we've forgotten is, our bodies evolved in tandem with the plants that offer an abundance of spices and herbs. These spices and herbs were used to make (often unpalatable) food palatable as well as for food preservation and cultural traditions. The distinction between what was considered "food" and "medicine" was not always so starkly drawn.

Today, however, as people reach for bland and salty processed foods, we see less use of culinary spices and more prevalence in the conditions these spices can actually prevent and treat. While this may not be a causal relationship, I do have a clear observation: We need the medicine of spices.

To compound the issue, holistic, integrative, or herbal medicine tends to be expensive and inaccessible to the general population. What was once a simple daily practice, herbal medicine has become the medicine of the elite, with fancy products in pricey bottles. And while there are many wonderful companies and products out there, herbal medicine does not need to be expensive or exclusive. In fact, the more you can taste and smell and touch and grind and sift the medicines you are using, the better. Backed by a plethora of scientific evidence supporting the beneficial properties of using herbs and spices for health, I am making the call for more people to use medicinal spices every day.

Finally, I want to say, this is the medicine of families, communities, and traditional cultures. A whiff of celebratory cardamom can conjure the joys of a wedding; the heady scent of fresh rosemary conveys a sense of elegance. While children sprinkle cinnamon in their hot cocoa, their grandparents can add it to a dinner dish to support cardiovascular health.

Spices are our perfect medicine. They are my daily tonic, my connection to past and present. They also bring joy to the food I prepare for my family. I invite you to integrate spices into your diet, and to enjoy the health-boosting deliciousness that they bring.

Bevin Clare

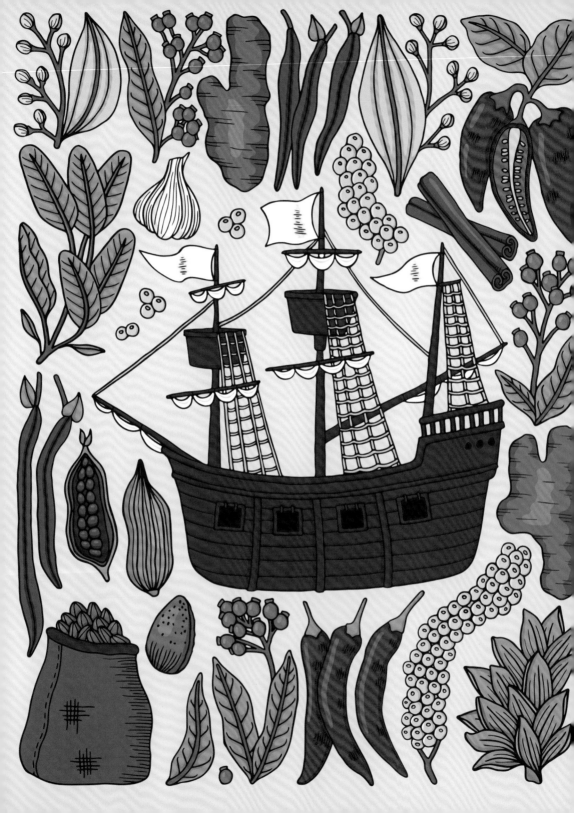

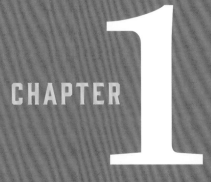

CHAPTER 1

Our Connection to Spices

Our senses are attuned to the taste, touch, and smell of spices. Across the globe, people have made use of spices as food flavorings, medicines, and even as valued cultural totems. And despite an ever-growing industry of synthetic flavors, we return again and again to spices for use as fragrant foods and as medicines.

THE GLOBAL SPICE TRADE

We have long been tantalized by spices. They have been more valuable than gold, the topic of wild lore, and the glories of great societies. They have incited us to cross vast oceans, fight wars, and seek treasures. Many of the most important trade routes in the world were developed for trading spices — specifically, among the Middle East, India, and China and their connections to Europe.

Look at a map of Europe and you'll see the lasting effects of the spice trade routes. Venice became a major port where ships sailed in with exotic ingredients from afar, such as ginger, cinnamon, and peppercorns. The Dutch and English competed to colonize areas of the globe that were rich in spices, and to establish trade routes to them. Spices played a significant role during the hundreds of years that European nations sought to colonize tropical countries — often extracting profit from these cultures without giving many benefits back, or causing harm and violence. Indeed, the desire for the flavors of rare spices has been powerful and often destructive.

Christopher Columbus bumped into North America when he was seeking a more efficient route to the Spice Islands — known as Indonesia today. But the New World does not offer the abundance of spices that were found in Asia or even Europe. The most favored herbs and spices brought from the Americas to Europe were vanilla, chili peppers, and allspice.

Today, the United States is the world's leading consumer of spices, and Asia is the largest producer. Some spices, like peppercorns, have become big business, and their centers of production have moved across the world from where the spice is native. A vast quantity of peppercorns (native to the Americas) are grown in Brazil; ginger (native to Asia) is grown in the Tropics.

One thing that has remained consistent over centuries is the relative expense of spices. The price tends to correlate to the difficulty of growing. Famously, the most expensive spice is saffron. Saffron is the stigma of the crocus flower, and it is incredibly labor-intensive to harvest. There are only three stigma in a saffron flower, and the harvesting has to be done by hand. Then, each tiny stigma must be dried to preserve its color and flavor. The second most expensive spice to harvest and buy is vanilla. Vanilla plants are in the orchid family and are notoriously difficult to grow and pollinate. The fruits (vanilla beans) of these delicate plants take a long time to mature, and they must be harvested at a precise time, requiring intensive cultivation and a lot of human labor.

Today, spices are grown around the globe. Most of them are cultivated in the tropics and are sold in large quantities in more temperate regions. While the United States, European Union, and Japan are leaders in purchasing herbs and spices, these countries grow very few of the spices on the global market. As our tastes become more global, our desire to have a greater diversity of spices available in our communities increases. Trends show increases in the purchase and consumption of spices around the world, regardless of economic or developmental status. Spices have become a truly global power in health and cuisine.

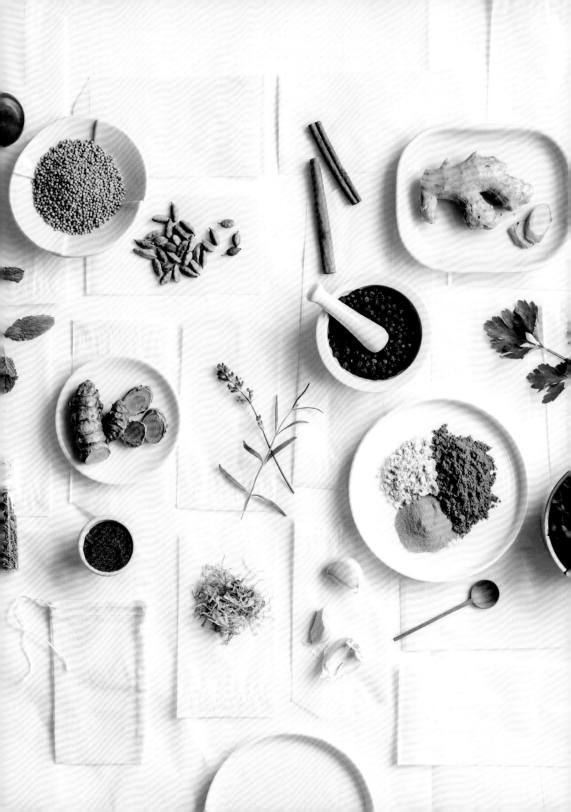

NATIVE SPICES

NORTHERN EUROPE AND EURASIA

Caraway (*Carum carvi*)
Celery seed (*Apium graveolens*)
Chives (*Allium schoenoprasum*)
Horseradish (*Armoracia rusticana*)
Juniper (*Juniperus communis*)
Mint (*Mentha* spp.)
Mugwort (*Artemisia vulgaris*)
Southernwood (*Artemisia abrotanum*)

MEDITERRANEAN

Ajwain (*Trachyspermum copticum*)
Anise (*Pimpinella anisum*)
Arugula (*Eruca sativa*)
Coriander (*Coriandrum sativum*)
Cumin (*Cuminum cyminum*)
Fennel (*Foeniculum vulgare*)
Hyssop (*Hyssopus officinalis*)
Lavender (*Lavandula angustifolia*)
Myrtle (*Myrtus communis*)
Nigella (*Nigella sativa*)
Oregano (*Origanum vulgare*)
Parsley (*Petroselinum crispum*)
Rosemary (*Rosmarinus officinalis*)
Rue (*Ruta graveolens*)
Saffron (*Crocus sativus*)
Sage (*Salvia officinalis*)
Savory (*Satureja hortensis*)
Sumac (*Rhus coriaria*)
Thyme (*Thymus vulgaris*)

AFRICA

Grains of Paradise
(*Aframomum melegueta*)
Kani pepper (*Xylopia aethiopica*)
Sesame (*Sesamum indicum*)
Tamarind (*Tamarindus indica*)

THE AMERICAS

Allspice (*Pimenta dioica*)
Annatto seeds (*Bixa orellana*)
Cacao (*Theobroma cacao*)
Chile pepper (*Capsicum* spp.)
Epazote (*Chenopodium ambrosioides*)
Lemon verbena (*Lippia citriodora*)
Mexican pepperleaf (*Piper auritum*)
Mexican tarragon (*Tagetes lucida*)
Nasturtium (*Tropaeolum majus*)
Oilseed pumpkin (*Cucurbita pepo*)
Paprika (*Capsicum annuum*)
Pink pepper (*Schinus terebinthifolius*)
Sassafras (*Sassafras albidum*)
Spilanthes (*Spilanthes acmella*)
Vanilla (*Vanilla planifolia*)

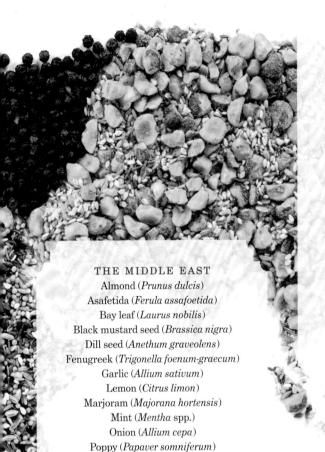

SOUTHEAST ASIA
Cloves (*Syzygium aromaticum*)
Cubeb pepper (*Piper cubeba*)
Ginger (*Zingiber officinale*)
Greater galanga (*Alpinia galanga*)
Kaffir lime (*Citrus hystrix*)
Lemongrass (*Cymbopogon citratus*)
Lesser galanga (*Kaempferia galanga*)
Lime (*Citrus aurantifolia*)
Long pepper (*Piper retrofractum*)
Mace and Nutmeg (*Myristica fragrans*)
Perilla (*Perilla frutescens*)

SOUTH ASIA
Basil (*Ocimum basilicum*)
Black cardamom (*Amomum subulatum*)
Black cumin (*Bunium persicum*)
Black pepper (*Piper nigrum*)
Cardamom (*Elettaria cardamomum*)
Cinnamon (*Cinnamomum
zeylanicum, C. verum*)
Curry leaf (*Murraya koenigii*)
Long pepper (*Piper longum*)
Turmeric (*Curcuma longa*)

THE MIDDLE EAST
Almond (*Prunus dulcis*)
Asafetida (*Ferula assafoetida*)
Bay leaf (*Laurus nobilis*)
Black mustard seed (*Brassica nigra*)
Dill seed (*Anethum graveolens*)
Fenugreek (*Trigonella foenum-graecum*)
Garlic (*Allium sativum*)
Lemon (*Citrus limon*)
Marjoram (*Majorana hortensis*)
Mint (*Mentha* spp.)
Onion (*Allium cepa*)
Poppy (*Papaver somniferum*)
Rose (*Rosa* spp.)
Tarragon (*Artemisia dracunculus*)

EAST ASIA
Cassia cinnamon
(*Cinnamomum cassia*)
Ginger (*Zingiber officinale*)
Lesser galanga (*Kaempferia galanga*)
Perilla (*Perilla frutescens*)
Sichuan pepper
(*Zanthoxylum piperitum*)
Star anise (*Illicium verum*)
Wasabi (*Wasabia japonica*)

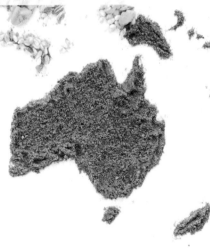

UNDERSTANDING THE PLANTS

When you enjoy the taste or smell of a spice you are experiencing something critical to the survival and health of the plant from which it was harvested. The aromatic compounds created by plants that we call spices serve many purposes beyond piquing our palate. They are part of plant communication and defense as well as part of a connection between related plants circling the globe.

Herbalists use the name "herbs" to refer to the medicinal parts of plants in a broad sense. When we look to herbs and spices for culinary use, we typically consider spices to be the seeds, flowers, bark, roots, buds, pollen, and fruits of plants, while we call the leaves herbs. Don't get too hung up on the terminology; they're all

plant parts, and wherever a plant concentrates its flavor we can harvest the part for medicine.

We can also harvest different spices at different times of growth from the same plant. As you may know, cilantro and coriander come from the same plant. We harvest the green leaves as cilantro, and when they mature and turn to seed, we have coriander. There are also optimal times to harvest plants for the best flavor. Vanilla, for example, can take up to nine months to mature, and then as soon as the plant turns golden-green, the unripe pods are harvested. Some spices, like cinnamon, can come from any number of different species and will range dramatically in flavor, medicinal properties, and cost. Each spice has its own characteristics to consider when using it. Some spices are best dried, others are best fresh; some are processed or smoked before use, and others are fermented.

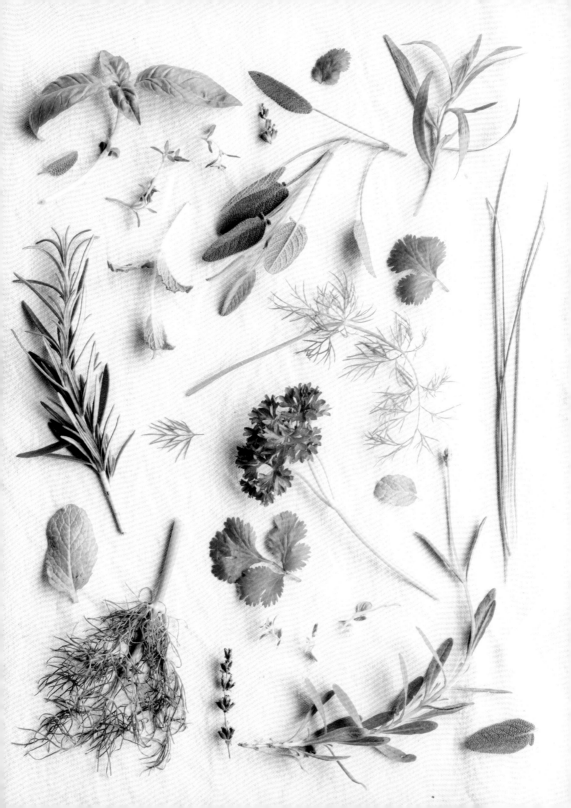

LEAVES AND AERIAL PARTS

ANGELICA (STEM)	EPAZOTE	PARSLEY
BASIL	FENNEL	ROSEMARY
BAY LAUREL	FENUGREEK	SAGE
CHERVIL	LEMONGRASS	SASSAFRAS
CHIVES (SCAPES)	MARJORAM	TARRAGON
CILANTRO	MINT	THYME
DILL	OREGANO	

FLOWER

CALENDULA

CHAMOMILE

LAVENDER

SAFFRON (STIGMA)

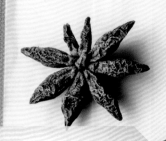

SEEDS AND PODS

ANNATTO

CARDAMOM

CELERY SEED

CHARNUSHKA/BLACK CUMIN

FENUGREEK

MUSTARD

POPPY

SESAME

STAR ANISE

FRUITS

ALLSPICE (BERRY)

ANISEED*

BLACK PEPPERCORN (BERRY)

CACAO (BEAN)

CAPSICUM PEPPER

CARAWAY*

CITRUS

CORIANDER

CUMIN*

DILL

FENNEL*

JUNIPER (BERRY)

MACE

NUTMEG

SUMAC (BERRY)

VANILLA (BEAN)

*THE DRIED FRUIT IS COMMONLY
REFERRED TO AS A SEED

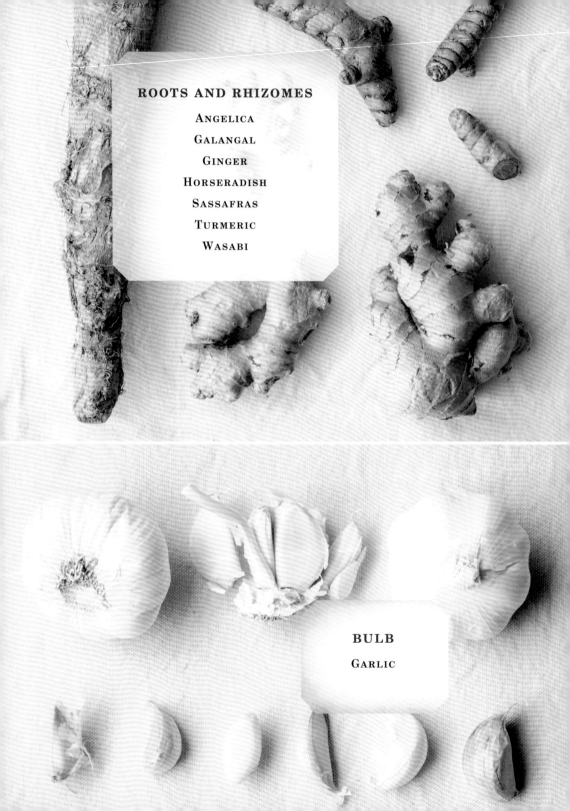

ROOTS AND RHIZOMES

Angelica

Galangal

Ginger

Horseradish

Sassafras

Turmeric

Wasabi

BULB

Garlic

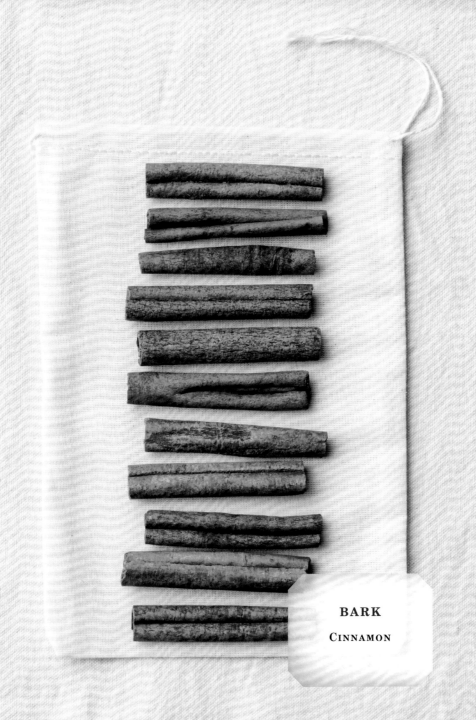

BARK

Cinnamon

PLANT FAMILIES

Plants, like all living organisms, are scientifically classified with their genetically similar relatives. When we talk about a plant, we are usually referring to a particular species. For example, when we talk about ginger, we are typically referring to *Zingiber officinale*. Sometimes there are varieties or hybrids within species to consider, such as in the mint family. In other cases, several spice species exist in one genus, such as in the citrus family.

Looking at spices as they are classified in plant families can offer some interesting insights. Plants in the same family often share phytochemical as well as physical characteristics. Look at *Apiaceae* (the carrot family) and you can see the similar leafy look of parsley and cilantro, while those in the mint family (*Lamiaceae*) all share the opposite-alternative leaf pattern you see in mint, basil, and sage. Knowing plants, and therefore spices, through a lens of their relationship to one another can also be applicable in cooking, as it can help us anticipate the characteristics of the aromatics and make something new or unfamiliar recognizable.

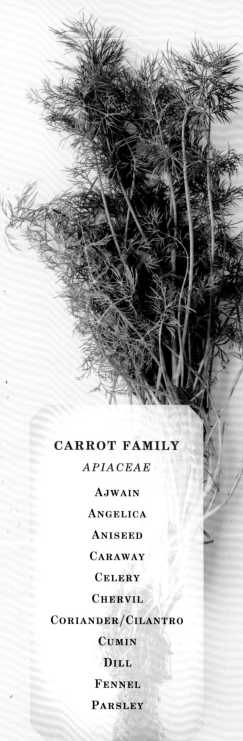

CARROT FAMILY
APIACEAE

AJWAIN

ANGELICA

ANISEED

CARAWAY

CELERY

CHERVIL

CORIANDER/CILANTRO

CUMIN

DILL

FENNEL

PARSLEY

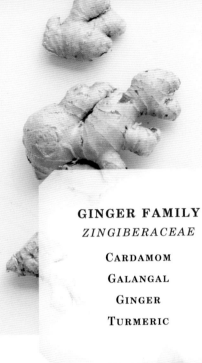

GINGER FAMILY
ZINGIBERACEAE

CARDAMOM

GALANGAL

GINGER

TURMERIC

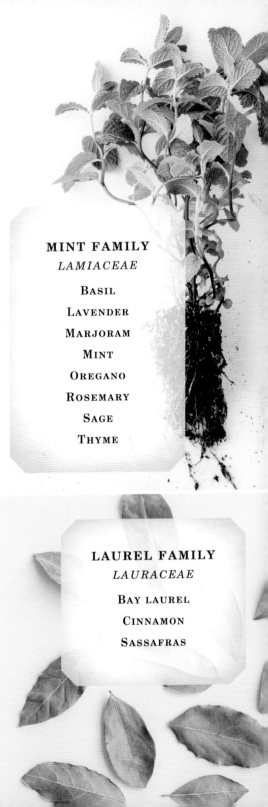

MINT FAMILY
LAMIACEAE

BASIL

LAVENDER

MARJORAM

MINT

OREGANO

ROSEMARY

SAGE

THYME

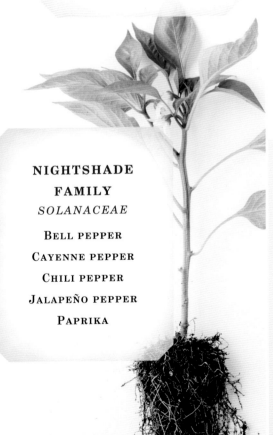

NIGHTSHADE FAMILY
SOLANACEAE

BELL PEPPER

CAYENNE PEPPER

CHILI PEPPER

JALAPEÑO PEPPER

PAPRIKA

LAUREL FAMILY
LAURACEAE

BAY LAUREL

CINNAMON

SASSAFRAS

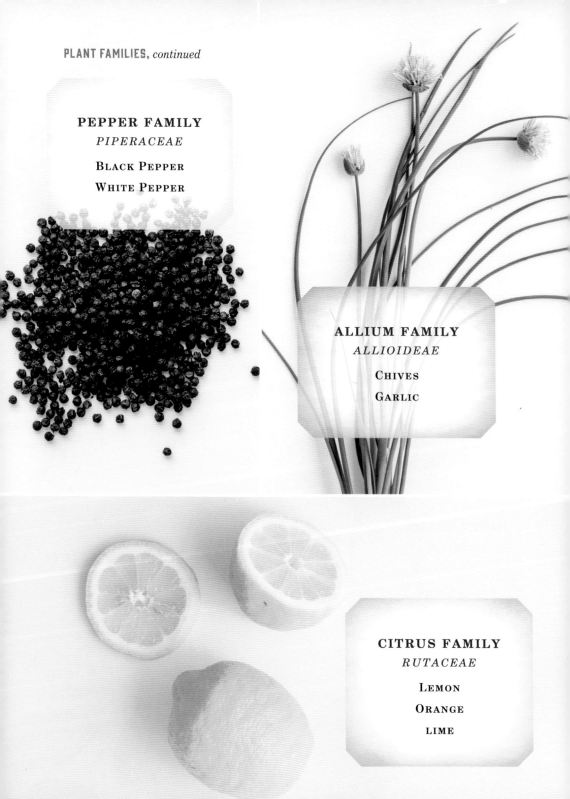

PEPPER FAMILY
PIPERACEAE

BLACK PEPPER

WHITE PEPPER

ALLIUM FAMILY
ALLIOIDEAE

CHIVES

GARLIC

CITRUS FAMILY
RUTACEAE

LEMON

ORANGE

LIME

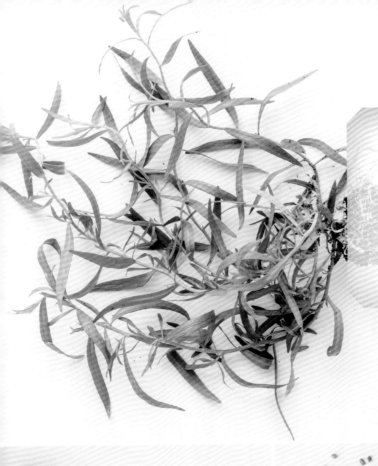

DAISY FAMILY
ASTERACEAE

CALENDULA

CHAMOMILE

CHICORY

TARRAGON

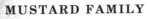

MUSTARD FAMILY
BRASSICACEAE

HORSERADISH

MUSTARD

WASABI

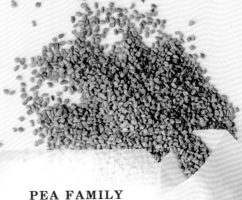

PEA FAMILY
FABACEAE

FENUGREEK

LICORICE

17

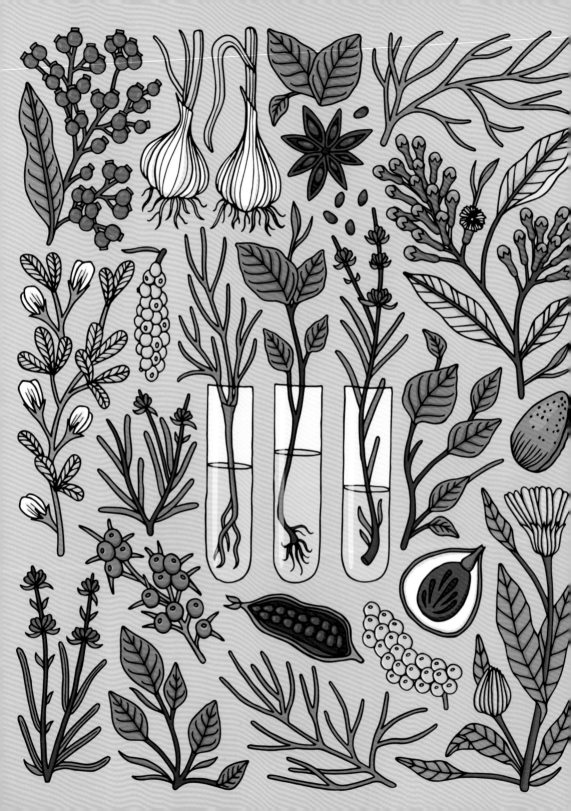

CHAPTER 2

How Medicinal Spices Work

Spices play a significant role in human health — a role that is vastly underestimated in Western medicine. At the bare minimum, spices have long been important in food preservation, as they inhibit the growth of undesirable bacteria and other pathogens. More importantly, spices offer a phytochemical diversity that contributes to the prevention, and even reversal, of a variety of common diseases.

SPICES IN
OUR DIET

PHYTOCHEMICAL
POWERHOUSES

The Mediterranean diet has long been touted for its health benefits — typically attributed to the high-quality fats, whole grains, fresh fish, and prevalence of fruits and vegetables. What is neglected in this discussion is the heavy reliance on fresh and dried herbs, like fennel, parsley, thyme, oregano, and nigella, that are so ubiquitous in the foods of the Mediterranean region. These spices (and others) offer abundant antioxidants, phytochemical diversity, and a broad profile of medicinal qualities.

The more we learn about the medicinal powers of spices, the more possibilities come into focus regarding use of spices for health. Abundant evidence supports the use of spices in our food for the prevention, and even possible treatment, of some of our most common health concerns, such as heart disease, arthritis, and even cancer. The possibilities of the therapeutic application of spices is also bolstered by the safety data we have amassed by consuming these plants regularly for thousands of documented years. Food plants are, fundamentally, very safe to eat, and it is nearly impossible to take an unsafe dose in culinary form.

And here's the best part: unlike some things we know we *should* be doing for our health but don't really *feel* like doing, consuming spices is enjoyable, affordable, and easy. We have an opportunity to fill our lives (and plates) with spices and find pleasure in their delicious medicine.

Spices are some of the most complex members of the plant world. One plant can have hundreds of different bioactive compounds. These different compounds can have a specific impact on human health and disease, and when you get the whole bundle together there can be all sorts of amazing synergy happening. Phytochemical power is the collective power of the many components that make up a medicinal plant. While we can understand the specific action of a specific compound, when you have all the components together in the whole plant, their interactions with one another are massively complex — and beneficial for us.

These plants use their phytochemical power not, in fact, for the sake of human enjoyment but rather for their own intra-species communication. In other words, the smells and tastes we love in spices are also essential aspects of the plants that are necessary for survival of the species. We are the lucky recipients of this plant chemistry, receiving the aromatic delights of the spice world. And while we enjoy the flavors of peppers or garlic or ginger, the health benefits extend beyond a bit of goodness in our bowl.

POLYPHENOL PROTECTORS

The group of phytochemical constituents that predominates in most medicinal spices are polyphenols. Polyphenols are a large group of compounds that are structurally diverse. There are a number of different subtypes of which you've likely heard, including flavonoids, isoflavones, flavonols, phenolic acids, coumarins, tannins, and lignans.

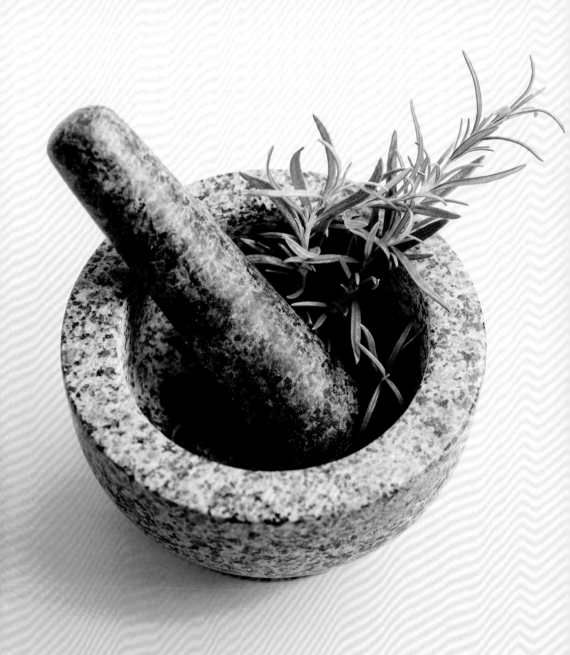

Aromatic plants such as rosemary (pictured here) are an integral part of the healthiest diets in the world. Rosemary plays a role in the significant health benefits of the Mediterranean diet.

Polyphenols are most famous for their antioxidant effects in the body, which are critical to maintaining good health. They contribute to optimal cell function and cellular maintenance and also play a role in decreasing inflammation. Some of these effects point to the anti-cancer and neuroprotective benefits of spices and medicinal plants. Antioxidants can have significant impact on conditions that involve inflammation, such as cardiovascular disease, type 2 diabetes, asthma, immune health, and infection. Polyphenols aren't found in spices alone; they are common in the plant world, but herbs and spices contain a relatively high level of polyphenols, especially phenolic acids and flavonoids.

ANTIOXIDANT AVENGERS

We've all heard that antioxidants are good for us, but it's important to understand the complexity of food-based antioxidants. A specific food may have tremendous antioxidant potential when it is sitting on a plate, but that doesn't necessarily indicate what will happen when it gets into your body. There are antioxidants that can survive or even potentiate (increase effectiveness) once inside the digestive system, directly impacting free radicals and other inflammatory substances in the body. Other antioxidants, however, are destroyed during digestion or are converted into something that has a different effect on the body.

As medicinal plants, spices can have a number of different effects on the body because of their diverse chemistry. An important point to note when using medicinal spices is that you aren't necessarily looking for the direct anti-inflammatory or antioxidant capacity of a plant. Instead, you

should focus on how the plant influences your endogenous (internal) processes and your body's ability to reduce inflammation and oxidation (the destruction of cells). Human beings have adequate internal systems to reduce inflammation and mitigate oxidation, but our lifestyles and diet, coupled with genetic propensities, make inflammation the root cause of nearly all chronic and degenerative diseases today. Medicinal spices can offer the necessary tools and chemical messengers to stimulate internal systems and, in turn, decrease inflammation.

RESEARCH ON MEDICINAL SPICES

A lot of research examining the impact of diet on the health of a population or an individual fails to take into account the impact of medicinal spices. Too often spices are considered flavoring agents rather than medicinal substances. So, how do we know that spices have specific effects in humans, especially when they are generally combined with foods that may have similar or overlapping effects?

The largest inhibiting factor to better understanding the action of herbs and spices on the body is a lack of funding for research on culinary spices. Typically, research is funded to address a major health epidemic or acute need, or it is based on the development of drugs. Spices, as such, cannot be patented or sold as drugs, so their earning potential and the subsequent available research funds are minimal. Companies can, however, develop what they call "natural products" that have a specific target, such as a toothpaste that reduces plaque buildup or a customized formula for joint inflammation. Or, they can isolate one or more individual constituents such as concentrated allicin from garlic. These strategies allow companies to sell products to the consumer at a much higher price than what you'd pay for the raw ingredients.

Additionally, plants can be difficult to study because of their multiple constituents (the hundreds of chemical compounds that are part of a plant), diversity in chemistry, and biological range depending on area of cultivation, season, and other factors. The use of medicinal herbs and spices can be highly seasonal, depending on whether fresh or dried ingredients are available and in what abundance, making research even more complicated. As a result, we really don't have a great variety or the highest quality of human data to assess the impact that seasonal or regional differences in plant chemistry have on human health.

What we can do is look at the chemistry of medicinal plants and observe their effect in humans, animals, or specific disease states. This type of research tends to be fairly clear and concise, so we can know exactly how turmeric affects individuals who are developing type 2 diabetes. But to understand how turmeric impacts an individual who eats it in their curry every day is significantly more complicated, and our methods of data-gathering and analysis coupled with a lack of funding make these answers to these important questions elusive. We *do* know there are positive effects, proven in research, to consuming spices regularly but we are still learning how and why these happen.

WHOLE-PLANT HEALTH

In nearly all cases, choosing a whole spice rather than an isolated extract is best for maintaining daily health and wellness. While it's much easier to study a single constituent than to study the complexity of a whole plant (never mind a spice blend!), in many cases the evidence doesn't necessarily support the isolation and concentration of these constituents over the use of the whole spice in food. As a result, we've wound up with a lot of studies on isolated constituents, a lot of patented products, and a lot of drug-like substances — and a paucity of studies that examine the long-term dietary use of whole plant medicinal herbs and spices.

Spices in their whole, natural form are delicious and dynamic. Consuming them eliminates the scientific guesswork of trying to figure out how a plant works and trying to extract those benefits to create something "better." Natural and whole spices used for health offer a variety of advantages you might lose with an isolate constituent. There's no point in extracting a specific constituent solely for its impact on circulation when the whole plant might also have benefits for resolving high cholesterol or hypertension.

SPICES AND DISEASE PREVENTION

Our use of spices tends to be based on culinary desires, traditions, and habits rather than a targeted consumption for specific disease prevention. Even in cultures where the general population consumes a lot of one

Spices, in realistic doses and in their food-based form, can be difficult to study because of their natural complexity. Thankfully, our bodies have long relationships with the plant world and know how to use plants in ways that benefit us.

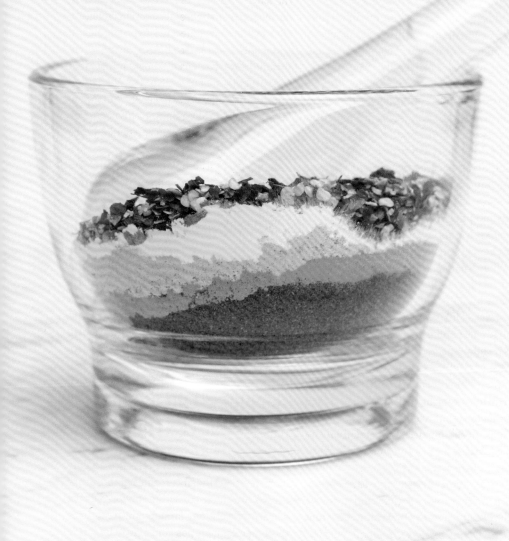

spice, such as garlic, it can be nearly impossible from a data perspective to tease apart the effects of garlic from the other foods one might be eating with it, such as olive oil or whole grains. The reality that one cannot live on spices alone makes it even more difficult to get a realistic picture of the impact of a commonly used culinary dose of a spice.

We can, however, study individual spices consumed in concentrated doses for a limited period. Nearly all the research on spices focuses on the effects of using a moderate to high dose over a limited period. It is easy to extrapolate from this research to hypothesize on the impact a spice might have at a smaller dose with less frequent use. Since we tend to use spices in blends coupled with other medicinal spices, small impacts can be amplified by consistent consumption of these tasty medicinal gems.

Research on medicinal spices and their impact on human health generally falls into four types of studies: in vitro, animal, human, and population studies.

IN VITRO STUDIES

In vitro studies are also known as "test tube research" and typically involve a specific human cell or group of cells that are introduced to a spice or an isolated component of a specific spice. These studies are cost-effective and efficient, but they omit considerable factors that would be present in real life, such as the impact of digestion on the spice and what form the spice would be in as it travels through the body. In addition, the concentration of spices as they appear in these studies is far higher than it would be in normal dietary consumption. Finally, in vitro studies often use a single isolated constituent from a medicinal spice. As spices are made up of hundreds of different constituents, it can be arbitrary or at least artificial to look at a single constituent. It can also significantly alter the medicinal effect of the plant. For example, a spice might have a constituent that is medicinally useful but not very bioavailable. In the same spice, there might be a few other ingredients that increase the bioavailability of the other constituents. Thus, the spice as a whole would be more medicinally active than any isolated part.

ANIMAL RESEARCH

Animal studies operate on the premise that other species (mice, specifically) are physiologically close enough to humans to allow us to learn about the effects of interventions on health and disease. Beyond the realm of studying potential toxicology of spices, the ethical aspects of animal studies are especially concerning with these substances that can be studied safely in humans. While there are models of animal research that do not harm the animal, this is the rare exception, unfortunately. Additionally, the administration of spices in animal research through artificial means, such as peritoneal injection instead of dietary consumption, brings up concerns in both applicability and ethics.

HUMAN CLINICAL TRIALS

Human research, especially double-blind placebo-controlled randomized clinical trials, is considered the gold-standard in looking at specific interventions in human health and disease. These studies can be controlled for other factors and allow us to learn as much as possible about a specific intervention using a variety of thoughtful

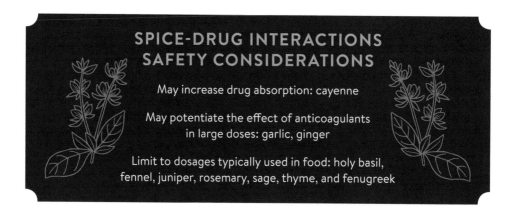

**SPICE-DRUG INTERACTIONS
SAFETY CONSIDERATIONS**

May increase drug absorption: cayenne

May potentiate the effect of anticoagulants
in large doses: garlic, ginger

Limit to dosages typically used in food: holy basil,
fennel, juniper, rosemary, sage, thyme, and fenugreek

data collection tools. Human clinical trials, while expensive, allow us to get a clear picture of how a specific spice might impact a specific aspect of health or disease at a specific dose with a specific preparation. What these trials don't do is gauge the overall general impact of consuming one or more spices dietarily over a long period of time.

POPULATION STUDIES

These studies tend to look a group, often a specific population, that shares a lifestyle or dietary trait. For example, a study might look at a group of seniors in a specific geographic region who consume a certain diet and compare it to others who consume a different diet. While it is possible to control for a variety of things that might impact data, such as socioeconomic status or race, the most we can hope to show with this sort of data is correlation. In the case of whether or not to consume a spice, correlation may be enough to convince us, but it does lack the specificity that clinical trials provide. That said, the use of the spices in population studies is much more representative of the

realistic day-to-day use of spices in dietary preparations.

SAFETY PRACTICES

Spices are incredibly safe. We have thousands of years of history to draw global data from regarding safety of culinary use. Most spices are used in relatively small quantities in cooking. I think of them more like concentrated foods than like drugs. Their complexity and versatility, coupled with humans' coevolution with aromatic plants, allows spices to offer the human body numerous benefits without creating any significant health risks.

SPICE-DRUG INTERACTIONS

It is, of course, critical to consider safety precautions of spices interacting with drugs. People all over the world use spices in their daily cooking while simultaneously taking various pharmaceuticals. Consider the pungent curries full of concentrated spices used in nearly all meals in the Indian subcontinent. This practice doesn't necessarily prove safety, but it does indicate that we are highly adaptable to concurrent use of spices and pharmaceuticals. And in some cases, there may even be benefits of using the two together. When a spice is used in its natural form there is a significantly reduced chance of an interaction or safety concern. For example, curcumin has been shown to have several potential drug interactions. However, this does not appear to extend to turmeric, which has a variety of different constituents and may not have the same monodirectional activity with the more multifactorial approach of a whole plant.

Spices, like other medicinal herbs, are less regulated than pharmaceuticals. Often, this means that they do not undergo the same sort of safety and toxicity analysis that a pharmaceutical would when being brought to market. Since spices are whole, natural substances and are more like foods than pharmaceuticals, this difference in rigorous testing is perfectly fine if you follow some simple rules when using medicinal spices. For a healthy adult who is not pregnant, or for a child, any of the spices in this book in a reasonable food dosage is within safety parameters.

AREAS OF CONCERN

Problems can arise in specific areas when using medicinal spices if you diverge from traditional dietary application or if you have additional health considerations. The first area of concern applies when medicinal spices are used in a preparation other than a food-based form, especially one that eliminates the ability to taste the spice when consumed, as in a capsule or tablet. Most spices have strong flavor and there is a reasonable

limit to how much we can tolerate. Often, the plants with upper limits in how we experience the flavor correlate to the stronger chemistry in those spices that shouldn't be consumed in large amounts. For example, seeds in the parsley family, such as cumin, coriander, anise, and fennel, are all strong-tasting, and it would be difficult to take a dose that could be problematic. However, if you take the same spices and concentrate them in an encapsulated version and you cannot taste the flavors, it would be possible to take more than a safe amount. The unsafe levels of any of these spices are extremely high, and the most likely side effects of a large dose are gastric distress or nausea.

The second area of concern involves people who have compromised kidney function or who are taking a pharmaceutical regimen with a narrow therapeutic range. In these cases, adding an abundant amount of spices to a bland diet may change the metabolism of certain pharmaceuticals; or, for someone with reduced kidney function, spices could be a slight irritant. In the case of reduced kidney function, there isn't an immediate need to avoid or limit the dietary use of medicinal spices, however, regular monitoring for at least the initial consumption period is recommended. For people taking a pharmaceutical with a narrow therapeutic range, such as antiepileptic medication or immunosuppressive medication, there should be some consideration of the consistent use of any recommended spices.

Another possible interaction occurs between anticoagulant pharmaceuticals and spices such as garlic and ginger. However, regular and reasonable dietary use of either of these spices should be just fine with appropriate monitoring.

Have you ever wondered why some spices are mild and others burn your tongue? Or why the smell of certain spices float through the whole house? The aromatic and flavorful aspects of herbs and spices are fascinating chemistry.

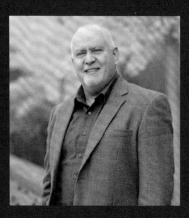

For **MICHAEL TIMS, PhD**, the mysteries of spices are held within the language of plants. Dr. Tims was lucky to grow up all over the world — in Thailand, Hong Kong, Germany, Romania, and Greece — and he was exposed to culinary traditions of each culture. Some of his fondest memories are of food, flavors, and aromas. He recalls cooking gumbo as a child with his mother and realizing that the combination of herbs and spices created a complexity of tastes and smells. The whole was greater than the sum of the parts.

As part of the Maryland University of Integrative Health, Dr. Tims thinks a lot about how medicinal plants develop the compounds that make them aromatic. We sat down to talk about how humans experience herbs and spices as scents and flavors.

Our sense of smell, says Tims, is influenced by the characteristics of the molecules responsible for odor. The key factors that allow us to smell them include how quickly the molecules volatilize (become airborne), how soluble they are in water or oil, and the acidity of food. Your genetics can also influence your sense of smell.

A molecule that we can smell is called a fragrance or odorant. Those molecules need to reach the olfactory system in the upper part of our nose. To do so, the molecular weight of these molecules needs to be very light. We have receptors in our nasal passages that are triggered by these molecules. Each olfactory receptor recognizes more than one odorant, and each odorant can be detected by several different olfactory receptors. We also know that the shape of a molecule is important and that when the molecule binds to a smell receptor, the receptor changes shape, which sends neural signals to the brain.

There are several theories out there on exactly how the perception of flavor and smell work at a molecular level. The shape of the molecule, its vibrational characteristics, its charge (polarity), and the tightness of a receptor binding can all influence the intensity of an odor.

THE SHORT AND LONG TAIL

So, let's compare the sweet, heavy scent of vanilla to the spicy, pungent smell of bay leaf. Starting with the basic structure, vanillin lends vanilla its signature sweet, perfumed, woody aroma. The molecular weight is relatively low and the molecules volatilize easily, filling a room with odor when they are cooked. The aroma of bay comes from eugenol. Comparing vanillin to bay is interesting as the eugenol in bay is built from the same basic structure, except eugenol has a short hydro-carbon-rich tail that gives it a stronger odor than vanillin. There is similarity in how the two molecules are structured, but the odor threshold of eugenol is lower than that of vanillin, which means you can smell it more easily and at smaller amounts. Eugenol's short hydro-carbon tail also creates a tighter binding with the odor receptor site as compared to vanillin, and explains why vanillin's odor is not as persistent as that of bay leaf.

Zingerone (found in ginger and mustard oil) has an even longer hydro-carbon tail connected to the basic vanillin shape, making it insoluble in water. It gives a rich, sweet, warm, and woody aroma. However, the presence of a carbonyl group in the tail means that the zingerone molecules tend to attract one another, preventing it from volatilizing. If it isn't volatizing, it isn't entering the air, and thus the aroma of ginger is less likely to fill a room as quickly with its aroma as vanilla.

Looking at an even heavier molecule, like capsaicin in cayenne, it also has a long, hydro-carbon-rich tail. The size of its tail limits the molecule's volatility, which means it is less likely to enter the air; and is one reason why cayenne doesn't smell so strong even though it certainly tastes strong. We can't always smell how spicy something is before we put it in our mouth! Next time you're cooking and the aromas are filling your nose, you might think about the shapes and characteristics of the molecules behind those wonderful smells.

1.

2.

1. Eugenol Molecule
2. Vanillin Molecule

PREGNANCY

Pregnancy creates a new set of circumstances to consider when using medicinal spices. Generally, spices in a food-based form are completely safe during pregnancy. However, many spices should be avoided in higher medicinal doses that exceed those typically used in food. When pregnant women are taking medicinal spices in dietary form there is usually a natural threshold that they will not exceed due to the strong flavor of spices. In a way, nature sets its own safety guidelines, assuming you can taste what you are consuming. That said, there are a number of spices that are appropriate and safe for pregnant women in generous culinary doses but should be avoided in large encapsulated doses, including turmeric, holy basil, fennel, juniper, rosemary, sage, thyme, and fenugreek.

The simple solution for safety in most situations is to use a variety of different medicinal spices each in a food-like dose. By choosing several different spices instead of one in a larger dose you'll find you do not have to use a high dose of any of them, and safety concerns are minimized. One exception may be cayenne or chili pepper, as even a small dose of these can increase absorption of pharmaceuticals. Keep in mind that individual absorption of pharmaceuticals can vary widely in the general population, with or without a spice like cayenne.

SPICE SYNERGY

When herbalists talk about synergy, we are referring to the compounded medicinal effects of using more than one botanical in a formula. Synergy is the interaction or cooperation of two or more substances to produce a combined effect greater than the sum of their separate effects. We experience this regularly with the food we eat, when a combination of foods creates a whole new flavor and texture to experience. Just think, it doesn't sound particularly exciting to eat a piece of bread, a bowl of tomato sauce, and some cheese — but how about a pizza!

Nearly every culture around the world has a long history of blending spices together. Common culinary spice combinations — like ginger and garlic or parsley and sage — are dynamic and often more palatable than one ingredient alone. That doesn't mean you can't use a single spice to make things more delicious — I do it all the time. But, when you blend spices together in a dish, the health-boosting possibilities are greater.

The concept of synergy can also be helpful if you are working with spices that may be less palatable but are desirable for their medicinal effects. For example, celery seed is effective in treating the accumulation of uric acid in someone who has gout. I'm sure there are some celery seed devotees out there, but most people would find this spice difficult to consume in large quantities. One possible solution is to combine other spices that are kidney tonics, such as parsley and sage, with spices that have a similar chemical composition to celery seed, such as anise, fennel, or coriander.

TO COOK OR NOT TO COOK

A number of factors can increase or decrease the medicinal effect of spices, and one big question is whether or not to cook them. Let me first say that the best way to use medicinal spices is simply to use them however you enjoy them. Don't overthink it; just use them in abundance.

That said, to address the question of cooking versus not cooking spices, we need to consider the plants. Some plants lend themselves naturally to being eaten raw. Herbs that are fresh and tender, such as basil, mint, dill, cilantro, and chives, are delicious straight from the garden. Other fresh herbs, such as thyme, rosemary, and sage, as well as roots and rhizomes, such as ginger and turmeric are tougher, and cooking these can increase bioavailability and improve the food's texture.

For dried herbs, whether you use them cooked or uncooked depends on preparation. Some of the herbs and spices that are especially leathery, like bay leaves and rosemary, should always be cooked and probably even removed from food before consumption (there's no danger in consuming them, but they are not easily digestible). Finely ground or powdered spices can be used in recipes or sprinkled on top of foods like a condiment. Any method of cooking that uses moisture will increase the polyphenol availability of a spice. This includes making soups, stews, casseroles, steaming, and sautéing. Dry-heat cooking, like grilling or roasting, tends to decrease the bioavailability, but even though the polyphenol levels are not as high with these methods, this is still a healthy way to get the benefits of spices.

For people who are not doing a lot of cooking or may be heating up pre-made meals, having a spice blend to sprinkle on top of your food is a tasty and easy way to gain the medicinal impact of spices every day. I keep a shaker full of the Everyday on Everything Blend (see page 116) on my kitchen table. The good news is, whether you cook herbs and spices or don't cook them, your digestion also increases the antioxidant effects of spices. I love it when people and plants work together!

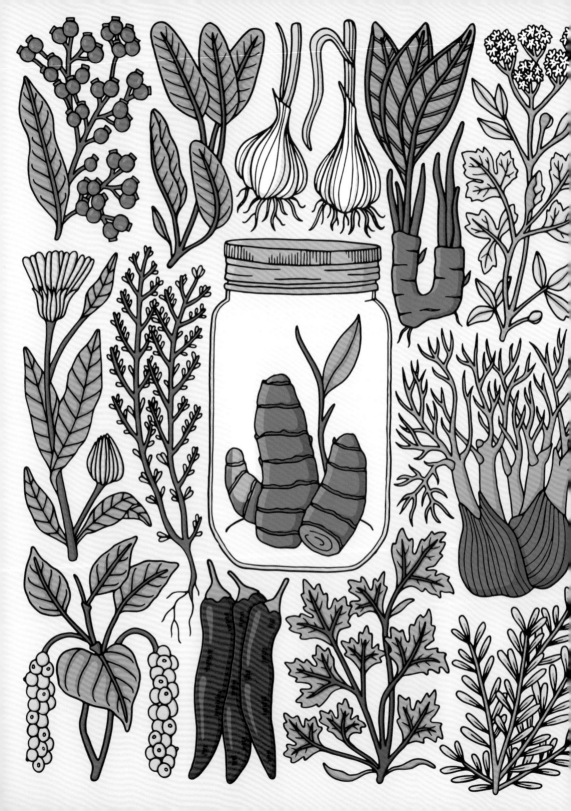

3

Creating Your Spice Apothecary

The 19 health-boosting spices in this chapter are fundamental to building your apothecary. Used for centuries by cultures around the world, these spices are accessible, versatile, and readily available, and they taste good. Their health benefits are also backed by clinical data. There are hundreds of other spices you may want to have in your apothecary, but these are a good start.

FRESH VS. DRIED

Spices can be used fresh or dried, with some forms being more commonly available in one form over the other. In parts of the world where fresh spices are abundant, you might find the opportunity to cook with fresh peppercorns or be lucky enough to play around with the vibrant yellow juice of turmeric. Dried spices offer convenience and a longer shelf life. They make it easy to keep spices close at hand year-round to add into everyday recipes.

FRESH MATTERS

Fresh herbs and spices can be found at a grocery store or farmers market — and in seasonal bounty in our gardens. A small plot or a series of pots can provide an ample supply of many wonderful herbs and spices. In almost any region in the world, you can cultivate at least 10 to 15 herbs and spices to use in cooking. Some of them can be available year-round even in temperate zones. I have pushed aside the snow to clip some rosemary or thyme, and it's a joy to harvest from a winter garden. If you have access to fresh herbs, you can learn to incorporate them into your daily meals in abundance. There are so many ways to include the most commonly found fresh herbs like basil, parsley, cilantro, ginger, garlic, or rosemary into every meal.

POWDERED VS. CUT AND SIFTED

Dried spices generally come either powdered or in small pieces commonly called "cut and sifted." In general, the hardier spices that come from roots, bark, and seeds are available as powder — like cinnamon, ginger, turmeric, and mustard. You can also get these spices fresh for use in infusing or for grinding or grating. Leafy spices are typically cut and sifted so that they can be easily integrated into food, and they keep longer in this form than when powdered. Use caution when buying powdered versions of the delicate parts of plants (leaves or flowers) as they will last only a short time due to the increased surface area.

BUYING

To find some of the less common spices or to purchase in large quantities, you'll want to look to herb and spice purveyors or markets where spices are sold in bulk (I've had good luck at Indian or Asian grocery stores). Another excellent place to buy spices can be the bulk bins at your local health food store, where you can buy any quantity by weight. Once you start cooking with herbs and spices, you'll find that the standard small jars from the supermarket chain are not enough, so it's worth it to buy in bulk for your most commonly used spices. Smaller quantities are fine for spices you use infrequently or in small amounts, such as cardamom, cayenne, clove, mustard, and nutmeg.

ONLINE

Spices can be purchased online through a variety of retailers, and they can vary widely in cost and quality. To ensure quality, purchase from a reputable vendor (see resources, page 156). A quality vendor will offer specific information on its website about each spice, including genus and species, and growing and sourcing. Inform

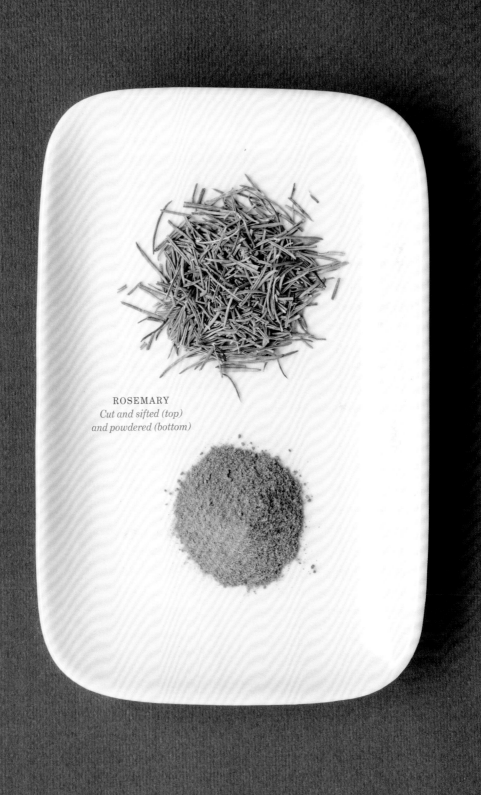

ROSEMARY
Cut and sifted (top)
and powdered (bottom)

yourself so you understand exactly what you are getting.

If you are looking for spice blends, seek out specialists in the type of cuisine you are preparing. For example, Indian curries can be made from hundreds of different combinations. If you buy from an Indian spice purveyor you may get more authentic or unique blends. When looking for the Moroccan spice blend Ras el Hanout, for example, you'll want to find a specialty spice purveyor who can offer the best quality and the freshest blend.

QUALITY AND FRESHNESS

The quality of spices can vary widely, and it can be difficult to know how to choose, especially since you can't open the package to smell or taste. For most spices, your primary quality concern is freshness. (In some cases, with rare spices such as saffron, there are concerns about adulteration and authenticity.) For leafy herbs, you should look for vibrancy of color. Dried leafy herbs, especially parsley and dill, tend not to stay fresh for long. If you tip the jar or bag and turn it around you can look for a bleached-out top layer where the herb has been exposed to light. If there is rich and vibrant color throughout, that's an indication of freshness.

Powdered spices tend to stay fresh for less time than whole spices, but the shortened lifespan needs to be weighed against the convenience factor. If I had to grind cardamom every time I wanted to use it, I probably would not use it as often. On the other hand, using whole spices whenever possible and grinding or powdering them in a mortar and pestle will offer a superior product — and it's a sensory delight.

When choosing a spice that has a wide range of varieties, such as chiles, cinnamon, or black pepper, the differences are primarily in flavor and aroma. However, if you are looking to address specific health conditions, there are therapeutic differences to consider in the genus and species of cinnamon (see page 53) and the type of chiles (see page 49).

STORING

Dried spices need to be protected from air, light, and heat. A beautiful display of light-filled spice jars in your kitchen offers less-than-ideal conditions for the spices' medicinal and culinary qualities. There are two simple ways to store dried spices in optimal conditions. One, store spices in glass or metal jars inside a pantry. There are all sorts of racks, organizers, and even magnets available for this method. The challenge with this method is that standard jars are pretty small for the amount of spices you'll want to have on-hand, and larger jars take up a lot of room on the shelf.

The second way, and my preferred method, is to use thick and sturdy zip-close bags for most spices. Some powdered spices, notably turmeric, do better stored in glass or in stiffer, thicker clear plastic bags that are used by spice companies. Alternately, some bulk spices are sold in foil bag, and these can be reused. Bags of spices take up far less room than jars and work well for both preservation and organization. I have a series of eight attractive little bins that hold my spices organized alphabetically into groups and slide neatly into a few shelves. You may have never noticed this, but there are a lot of spices at the beginning of the alphabet. Of my eight bins, I use half of them for As, Bs, and Cs!

If you have the space, most spices, especially those from leaves and flowers, will last longer and stay fresher if they are stored in the fridge or freezer. That said, many spices (especially those from roots, seeds, and barks) last a very long time. I remember going through my grandmother's spice cabinet and finding spices in small cardboard boxes that were at least 40 years old, and they still had aromatic and recognizable flavors — although I would certainly recommend using something much fresher for health and cooking!

Storing fresh herbs can be a little trickier. Ideally, you want to use fresh herbs quickly before they go bad. To make leafy fresh herbs last, store them with the cut part of the stalks in a small cup of water in the fridge — just a bit of water will do; don't let the leaves themselves touch the water. Basil, mint, parsley, dill, and cilantro do well this way, although it is important to change the water daily. Alternatively, you can wrap a small piece of damp paper towel or cloth around the stalk ends and store the herbs in a plastic bag in the fridge — just be careful not to bruise delicate basil or mint.

Herbs with more leathery textures, such as sage, thyme, bay, and rosemary, need less water to stay in good shape and can be stored in the produce drawer in your fridge either in or out of a bag. Discard fresh herbs if they become slimy or smell bad, but if they simply dry out inside your fridge there is no reason you can't use them as you would a dried herb.

Fresh roots such as turmeric or ginger tend to last much longer than the leafy parts of a plant. Ginger will last for several weeks in the fridge; and it's okay to slice off a bit of mold if it grows on the cut end and continue using the rest of the root.

THE DAILY DOSE

So, how much of a spice do you need every day? One of the primary reasons I was inspired to write this book is that people (including health practitioners) don't know how much a healthy daily dose is in culinary form. You might hear that you are supposed to take two grams of turmeric, so you go out and buy turmeric powder pills to swallow. For each of the 19 spices in the apothecary here, I have provided my clinical recommendations for a simple daily dose. The dosages are in both culinary measurements (like teaspoons) as well as in metric weight (grams).

Knowing proper dosages allows you to use spices in a more affordable and accessible way. While clinical studies and supplements measure spices in grams, it can be hard to know what four grams of garlic looks like in your kitchen. Here you have both, so you can inform and empower yourself to use spices for health.

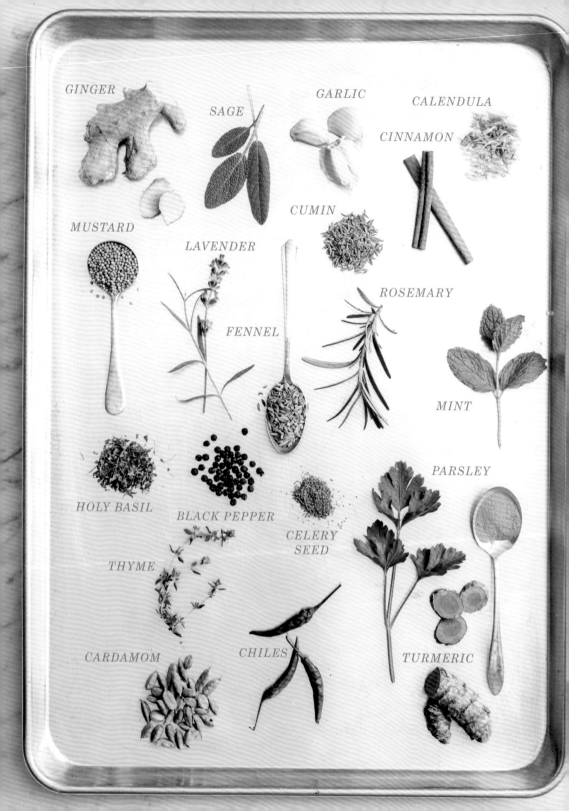

19 SPICES FOR EVERYDAY USE

It would be nearly impossible to compile all the spices used in food and medicine around the globe. People have traditionally used what is available in their geographic region. More recently in human history, we have gained access to hundreds of different spices and thousands of blends. Each spice has its own medicinal action.

I think of everything in my spice jars as spices. While we technically call the leaves of a plant *herbs*, I use the term *spices* to refer to any part of the plant that we harvest to use medicinally. The 19 spices we focus on in this apothecary are tasty and easy to find, and have proven health benefits. For practical use, these spices meet the following five criteria:

- Widely available and accessible in stores and through online retailers

- Affordable

- Used extensively in cuisines around the world

- Have an extensive history of use as medicine

- Show scientific evidence of health benefits through high-quality human clinical research

BLACK PEPPER

PIPER NIGRUM

Daily dose:
¼ teaspoon (1 gram) powdered

Black pepper is so common it can almost be overlooked as a healing spice. It sits on tables around the world and has the ability to bring out flavors and add a bit of a kick. While pre-ground pepper is widely used, its taste pales in comparison to the aromatic and tantalizing flavor of freshly cracked peppercorn.

In cooking, consider adding black pepper to a creamy or otherwise heavy meal. It can enhance other flavors in the dish and benefit digestion. Black pepper is also easily cracked right over the plate onto food. While other spices need heat from cooking to bring out their flavors and enhance bioavailability, black pepper can be added right to your dish.

Medicinally, black pepper is used to increase digestive fire and increase the bioavailability of other medicinal plants and their constituents minerals. Extracting vitamins and minerals from some foods can be tricky business, especially with any sort of digestive impairment or inflammation. Using black pepper might assist your body in getting what it needs from the healthy foods you are eating.

If you are looking to maximize your calcium absorption, for example, black pepper can help your body absorb minerals from greens and dairy into your bones. A noted example is the increase in bioavailability of curcumin in turmeric when they are consumed together. It's not a bad rule of thumb to put a bit of black pepper in just about any savory recipe you are making. Black pepper is also nice in some sweeter spiced foods that have a kick from cinnamon or cloves, such as chai, where it is a central ingredient.

BLACK PEPPER SPICE BLENDS
- Everyday on Everything Blend
- Fennel Dukkah Blend
- Green Goodness Blend
- Peppery Synergy Blend
- Reminds-Me-of-Pie Blend
- Warming Digestive Blend

BLACK PEPPER RECIPES
- Cinnamon Apple Oat Bake
- Cinnamon Spice Jellies
- Comfy Compote
- Dukkah Roasted Vegetables
- Green Goodness Dressing
- Heart Synergy Fudge
- Herby Gravy
- Spicy Virgin Bloody Mary
- Spicy Wonder Gingerbread

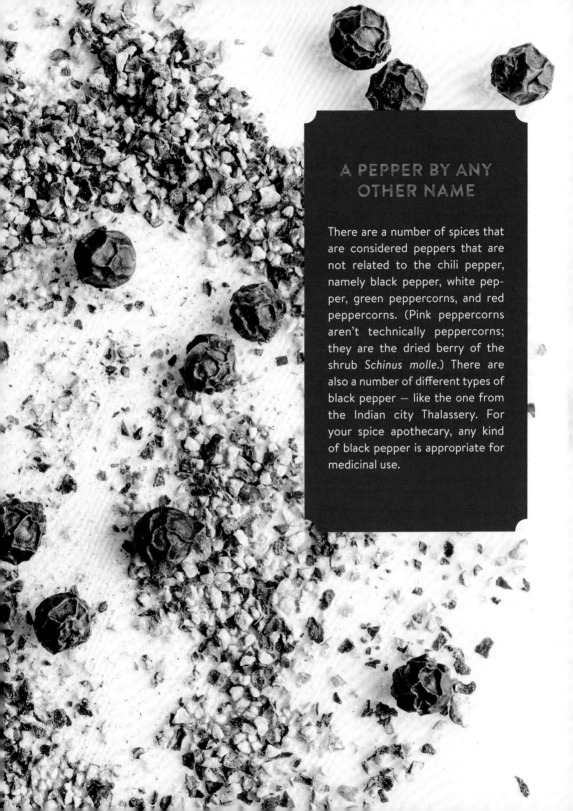

A PEPPER BY ANY OTHER NAME

There are a number of spices that are considered peppers that are not related to the chili pepper, namely black pepper, white pepper, green peppercorns, and red peppercorns. (Pink peppercorns aren't technically peppercorns; they are the dried berry of the shrub *Schinus molle*.) There are also a number of different types of black pepper — like the one from the Indian city Thalassery. For your spice apothecary, any kind of black pepper is appropriate for medicinal use.

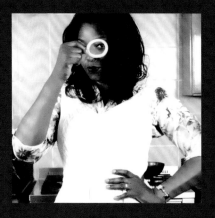

FUNKE KOLEOSHO is an award-winning cookbook author and food blogger who champions New Nigerian Cuisine with inspiring and delicious recipes. She is also a font of knowledge on traditional Nigerian spice combinations used for both culinary and medicinal purposes.

According to Funke, food is seen as medicine in Nigerian culture. While some herbs and spices are used medicinally in teas and tinctures, others (like ginger, garlic, turmeric, and basil) are added to soups, stews, and porridge to treat common ailments as has been done for thousands of years. Funke says that the most common medicinal herbs and spices used in Nigerian cooking include basil, chives, lemongrass, turmeric, garlic, ginger, and cloves. But there are also a variety of others that are lesser known and equally as beneficial.

Scent-leaf (*Ocimum gratissimum*) is an African native in the same genus as other basils and is known as Efinrin in Yoruba. One of its other common names is "clove basil," which is interesting, as it contains the sub-

in large levels in cloves. It's used fresh or dried and imparts a different flavor than many of the others in its genus because of its unique chemistry.

Bitter leaf (*Vernonia amygdalina*) is somewhere between an herb and a vegetable and is used to make a popular soup, stew, or sauce called ofe onugbu. The leaves, true to their name, are very bitter and typically prepared by rubbing them together under water to reduce some of the bitterness and then made into stew. Botanically, the plant is in the daisy/aster family, along with many other medicinal plants, such as echinacea, calendula, and chamomile. This huge plant family contains many food and medicine members but almost no spices (tarragon is the exception!) which makes bitter leaf even more interesting.

Grains of Selim (also commonly known as kani pepper) are both a spice and a medicine common to central Africa. They are fruits of the *Xylopia aethiopica* tree, a large evergreen tree in the Annonaceae family (sharing a family relation with soursop, custard apple, and the American pawpaw). The dried fruits have a musky odor that people compare to black pepper.

African nutmeg (also known as calabash nutmeg or Jamaica nutmeg) is the seed of the fruit from the *Monodora myristica* tree (also in the Annonaceae family). During the times of the slave trade, this tree was transported by seed to the West Indies. The seeds are similar to nutmeg (and are used interchangeably with nutmeg) but have many more medicinal applications.

Funke's Black Soup

Made with basil and a pepper sauce base, this medicinal soup is given to new mothers and people recovering from illness. You can alter the ratio of ingredients to your preference.

1 small chili pepper, seeded and chopped (more or less to taste)

2 medium onions

2 medium tomatoes

6 cloves of garlic

1 teaspoon fresh grated ginger

1 tablespoon palm oil

1 cup packed fresh basil leaves

2 cups cooked chicken pieces

4 cups chicken stock

Salt

1. Combine the chiles, onion, tomatoes, garlic, and ginger in a blender and blend until smooth. Heat the palm oil in a large saucepan, add the chile mixture, and cook over medium-low heat.

2. Meanwhile, blend the basil leaves in the blender until a smooth paste forms. Set aside.

3. Add the chicken and the chicken stock to the saucepan. Cover and simmer, stirring often, until the sauce is reduced to half its original volume. Season with salt to taste. Stir in the basil paste and let simmer for 3 minutes. Serve warm.

CALENDULA

CALENDULA OFFICINALIS

**Daily dose: 2 teaspoons (0.5–1 gram)
fresh flower petals**

Calendula likely isn't in your spice cabinet but it is widely used in herbal medicine. The brilliant yellow and orange petals of this flower are slightly bitter and saline. They add a gorgeous brightness to your cooking, along with a powerful medicinal benefit. Calendula ranks high on my list of favorite herbs and spices for its ability to heal damaged tissue. While there are many uses for topical application in herbal medicine, calendula's tissue-healing properties are wonderful for the gastrointestinal tract.

Calendula has great cultural significance in many places in the world. It was commonly used in Greek and Roman times for various rites and practices, and it plays a key role in ceremony and tradition in many Latin American and South American countries, including in the Dia de los Muertos celebrations, alongside its close relative Tagetes, another marigold. I once visited a cemetery in the south of Chile where every grave was turned into a flower bed for calendula, which demonstrates the great cultural significance of this plant.

If you are using dried calendula flowers or petals, it is best to use them whole because they degrade quickly when ground, and even whole dried calendula will begin to lose its vibrancy within a year or two. If you have fresh calendula in your garden, you can use the petals liberally in salads. It also makes a wonderful sunshine-colored infused oil. If you grow calendula, you can snap off the flower heads each day and add the petals into a jar of olive oil, allowing it to infuse throughout the growing season. The bright oil can be used for both medicine and as a base for marinades and salad dressings. It can be a pretty and powerfully antioxidant background for whatever flavorful herbs you might want to add in.

You can use dried calendula in cooking as you'd used dried thyme or rosemary, grinding or chopping it finely just before use. Dried petals can be added to soup or stews; the flavor is palatable and mild.

CALENDULA SPICE BLEND
- Green Goodness Blend

CALENDULA RECIPE
- Green Goodness Dressing

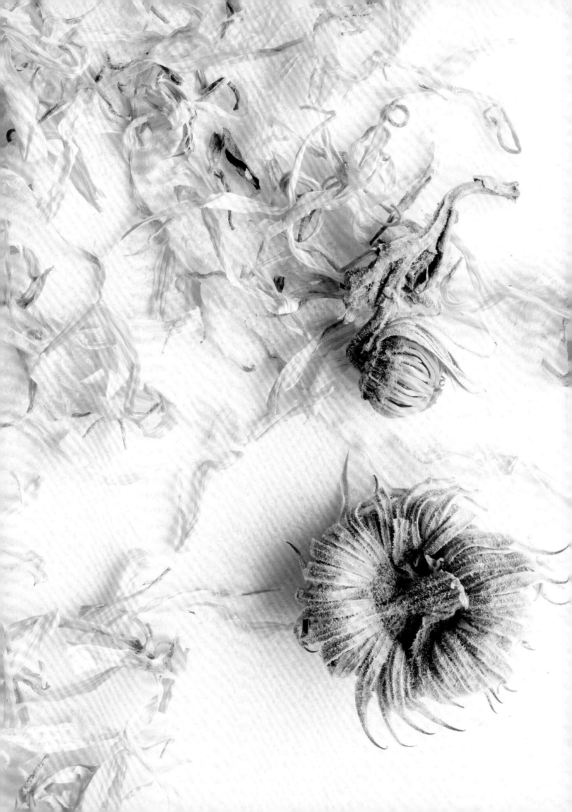

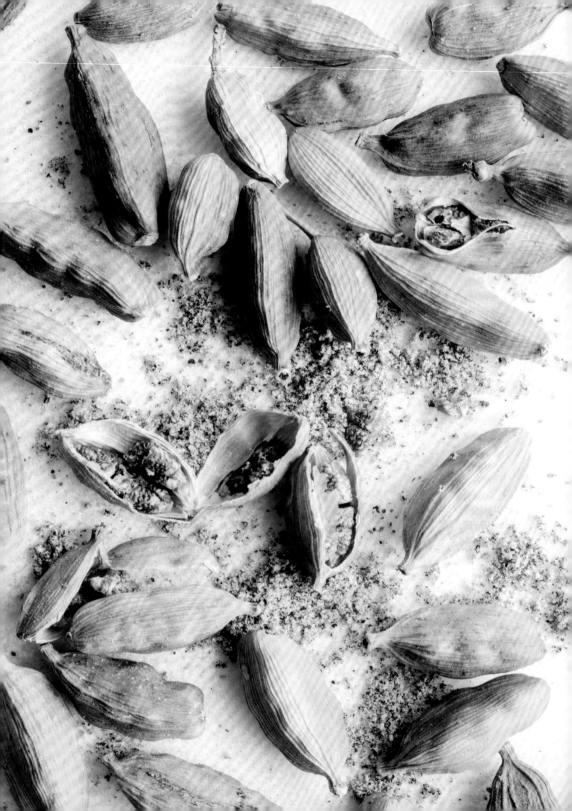

CARDAMOM

ELETTARIA CARDAMOMUM

Daily dose:
¼ teaspoon (0.8 grams) powdered

You'll find cardamom in a wide variety of traditional spice blends, especially in Indian cuisines. You may have come across cardamom in your tea mug if you've had chai. It's also a popular flavor in coffee in the Middle East.

This spice is native to India and Sri Lanka and is a member of the ginger family. Perhaps you can smell some similarities between the two? The cardamom plant might surprise you botanically with its quirky flowers and seed pods. Unlike ginger and turmeric, which have showy flowers atop green stalks, cardamom plants send out small, creeping branches along the ground, where modest flowers eventually turn to ripe pods. Cardamom is one of the most expensive spices in the world due to slow growth and small production of its precious pods. When purchasing cardamom, it can be tempting to buy the powder, but it degrades quickly and will last less than a year once ground. It's best to purchase the whole pods and grind them in a grinder or a mortar and pestle when you are ready to use them.

Cardamom has a mix of sweet and gently spicy flavor, although it can easily become overpowering when freshly dried. I once purchased a large bag of cardamom when I was traveling, and even after it was sealed and bagged in a half-dozen bags, I still had to leave it in a closet at night so I wouldn't be overwhelmed by the scent! It is a wonderful herb for digestion and is an appropriate substitute for ginger, for those who find ginger too spicy or the flavor of turmeric too strong. It's a nice spice to incorporate into a heavy or creamy dish, especially a dessert, as it can help with digestion. When using cardamom, a little goes a long way, so start small.

CARDAMOM SPICE BLENDS
- Reminds-Me-of-Pie Blend
- Warming Digestive Blend

CARDAMOM RECIPES
- Cinnamon Apple Oat Bake
- Cinnamon Spice Jellies
- Comfy Compote
- Spicy Wonder Gingerbread

CELERY SEED

APIUM GRAVEOLENS

Daily dose: ¼ teaspoon (1.5 grams) seeds

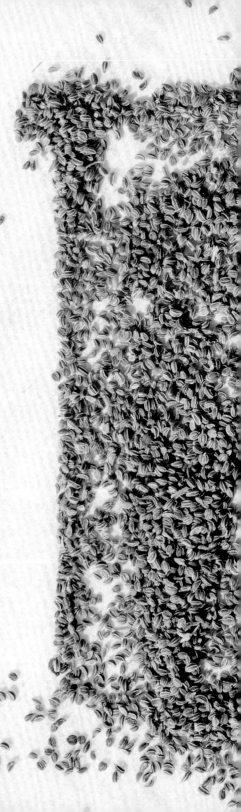

Celery seed is not the most common or beloved spice in the apothecary, and it can be a bit difficult to take in large quantities in food-based form. But it acts as a kidney tonic and can be used effectively with other kidney health herbs, like parsley, to leverage their synergy.

Celery seeds have a strong savory flavor and work best when used in robust and rich foods. The small seed should be used whole, as crushing them releases the more bitter elements. Celery seeds can be added liberally to oil-and-vinegar salad dressings or mayonnaise-based recipes, such as a potato salad or chicken salad. Celery seeds are also easily added to soups and stocks while simmering. They're also good in meatballs and meatloaf (you can use them as you would use fennel seeds).

CELERY SEED BLEND

- Seed Blend

CELERY SEED RECIPES

- Parsley Pesto
- Roasted Eggpant with Garlic Yogurt

CHILE PEPPERS

CAPSICUM SPP.

Daily dose: fresh, dried, or powdered; a little goes a long way

When we think of chiles, we might think of some of the spiciest cuisines in the world, from Southeast Asia, China, Sub-Saharan Africa, and India. It's easy to forget that chiles are a New World food, originating in South America, and that before chiles made their way out of the Americas and around the globe, these other regions used things like mustard, wasabi, and the mouth-numbing Szechuan peppercorn. Chiles were adopted into all of these cuisines by the late 1700s, which seems relatively recent when you consider their centrality to these regions and the diets of the peoples.

Today, chiles are used fanatically in a variety of sweet and savory foods around the world. Chiles grow best in tropical areas and can be grown year-round. Many chiles are easiest to use when fresh. Chiles are also commonly used to preserve foods against the effects of heat, especially in areas without refrigeration. Some people steer clear of chiles for fear of spiciness. But there are many different kinds of chiles and, while they are closely related, they are incredibly diverse in heat scale, color, flavor, and versatility.

CULTIVARS AND VARIETIES

All peppers, including bell peppers, are in the genus *Capsicum* (this does not include peppercorns, which are in a different family altogether). There are five major species of cultivated peppers in the genus *Capsicum*, and there are so many variations and cultivars it is difficult to create a definitive list. It's estimated that upwards of 50,000 pepper varieties exist today. Some of the most common peppers are in the *Capsicum annuum* group. These include bell peppers, sweet peppers, serrano peppers, cayenne peppers, paprika, and jalapeños. Another popular species is *Capsicum chinense*, which includes habaneros, scotch bonnets, and some other extremely spicy ones!

One of my favorite mild yet flavorful chiles is the ancho chile, commonly used in Mexican cooking. The ancho chile is a dried ripe poblano with a low heat level and a rich, deep, slightly smoky flavor. One of the many reasons I love it is that you can use it in large quantities to add medicinal benefits to a family-size meal without adding heat. When I make a pot of soup or chili, I will add a half-cup or more of ancho chili powder to create a rich, red gravy full of medicine. If spicy foods don't agree with you, try the ancho chile.

If you aren't afraid of spice, you can use hotter chiles. Powdered cayenne is great for sauces; just be sure to ease into it and use small amounts at first. It's always easy to add more spice to your dish but hard to take it out! You can also try adding jalapeños to your cooking — be sure to remove the seeds and slice the peppers finely. You may want to wear gloves when handling spicy chiles, as the oils can burn your skin and be painful if you touch your eyes, mouth, or nose. Also, note that chiles are nightshades; if you are sensitive to plants in the nightshade family you may not tolerate chiles well.

CIRCULATION AND SATIETY

Chiles are used to increase circulation and to increase the bioavailability and impact of other spices. If you have eaten spicy chiles no one needs to tell you that they get things moving in your body, as you sweat and feel the effects. The most widely used medicinal chili is cayenne, which is used both topically and internally. Topically, it's used to aid in local pain relief, and there is some research supporting its ability to reduce systemic pain. Cayenne can aide sluggish digestion and can also help move "stuck" things in the body — intestinal, respiratory, or even women's health problems. A midwife I know suggests a spicy meal for mothers who are waiting to go into labor — a great example of moving things along!

The addition of chile pepper to the diet may also change the way we experience fullness and even help decrease the amount we eat before feeling full. One study determined that red chili pepper and its constituent capsaicin have a positive effect on satiety (the feeling of being full during or after eating). People were given doses of chile pepper in their meals and then logged their hourly sense of satiety, fullness, hunger, and desire to eat. The results showed that red chili pepper consumption reduced hunger and increased satiety.

CHILI SPICE BLENDS
- Everyday on Everything Blend
- Mint and Chile Blend
- Not Necessarily Spicy Chili Blend

CHILI RECIPES
- Funke's Black Soup
- Garlic Spread
- Heart Healthy Hummus
- Herby Gravy
- Medicinal Miso Soup
- Minty Yogurt Spread
- Red Chili Pozole
- Spicy Virgin Bloody Mary

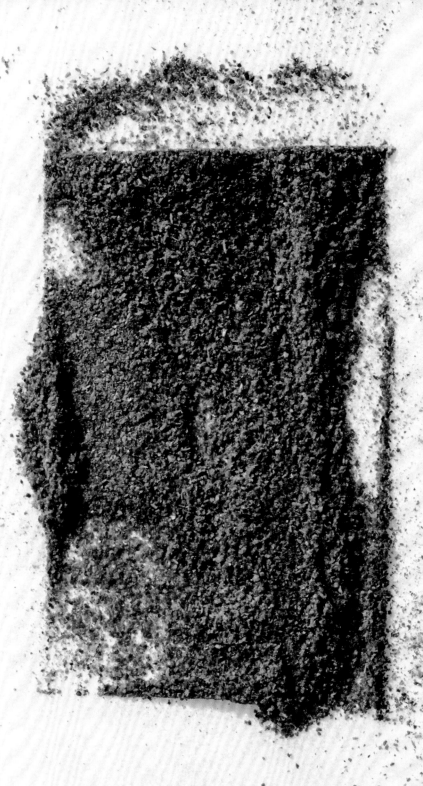

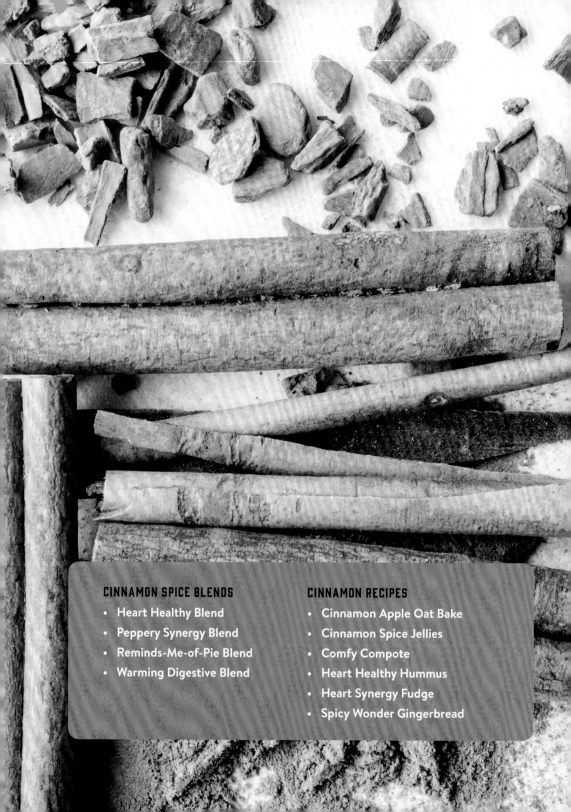

CINNAMON SPICE BLENDS

- Heart Healthy Blend
- Peppery Synergy Blend
- Reminds-Me-of-Pie Blend
- Warming Digestive Blend

CINNAMON RECIPES

- Cinnamon Apple Oat Bake
- Cinnamon Spice Jellies
- Comfy Compote
- Heart Healthy Hummus
- Heart Synergy Fudge
- Spicy Wonder Gingerbread

CINNAMON

CINNAMOMUM SPP.

Daily dose:
½ teaspoon (1.3 grams) powdered

Cinnamon is one of the oldest and most well-known spices. There are four commonly available types of cinnamon, and they can be quite different in taste, chemical composition, and medicinal action. All come from the inner bark of several Southeast Asian tree species from the genus *Cinnamomum* in the Lauraceae family.

Traditionally, cinnamon has been used for conditions of the digestive tract and the respiratory tract. More recently, it has also been employed for blood glucose management, diabetes, and inflammation. If you want to use cinnamon for prevention or therapeutics, a food-based dose of 1 to 2 grams per day offers significant health benefits and is palatable and easy to take. Sprinkle a half-teaspoon on top of your morning oatmeal, toast, yogurt, or applesauce.

When choosing a cinnamon, you'll want to consider the aroma and flavor as well as the coumarin content. Aroma and flavor are personal preferences and may depend on the type of preparation you are using, but the higher-quality cinnamons can be much more potent and aromatic.

Coumarin is a naturally occurring chemical compound found in numerous plants, including cinnamon, peppermint, celery, sweet clover, lavender, and carrots. The use of coumarin as a food additive was banned by the United States Food and Drug Administration in 1954, based on reports of hepatotoxicity in rats (and potential hepatotoxic effects in humans). While the small to moderate amounts of coumarin present in some cinnamon isn't a problem with occasional use, it can be a concern when you are using a regular therapeutic dose.

CULTIVARS AND VARIETIES

The most common species you'll see for sale in North America is *Cinnamomum cassia*. This spicy and strong-tasting cinnamon typically comes from China and makes up at least 50 percent of available cinnamon on the market. It comes from a harder tree bark and contains higher levels of coumarin than softer-bark varieties. In typical food doses, coumarin in cinnamon isn't anything to be worried about, but in some parts of the world, such as Germany, there is a ban on *Cinnamomum cassia* because of its coumarin levels. If you intend to take large doses for health, it is best to choose a different species of cinnamon.

If you are eating a little cinnamon here or there to enjoy the flavor, the *C. cassia* species is fine. But if you are taking cinnamon in regular, therapeutic doses, such as the recommended 1 to 2 grams per day, you'll want to use the safer, more medicinal species, *Cinnamomum verum*.

All of the commercially available species of cinnamon have been studied for use as medicine, mainly in their application for blood glucose regulation. *Cinnamomum verum*, or "true" cinnamon, has shown the most clinical promise, although all cinnamon demonstrates some medicinal activity. This cinnamon has a soft, thin bark and is known for its delicate and complex flavor as well as its sweetness. A quality spice purveyor will carry a variety of cinnamons, and you can ask for the species you are looking for.

CUMIN

CUMINUM CYMINUM

Daily dose:
½ teaspoon (1.5 grams) powdered

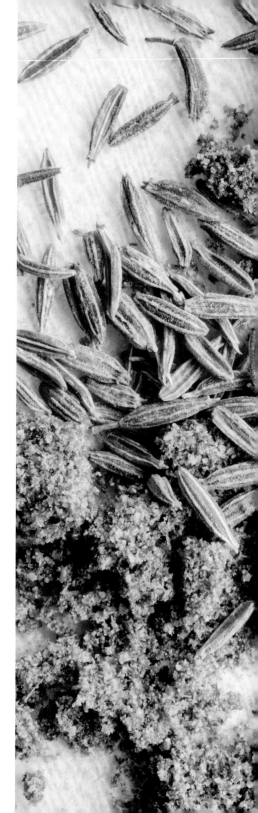

Another member of the *Apiaceae* (or parsley) family, this humble seed is used whole or ground and has an earthy flavor that becomes pronounced when dry-toasted (whole seed) or when added into hot oil. Both of these practices are common in traditional preparations using cumin. Cumin is often combined with other aromatic spices in sauces and curries, in either a whole-seed or ground form, most notably as a primary ingredient in garam masala, a spice blend central to Indian cuisine. Although related, black cumin (*Carum persicum*), used commonly in the Middle East, is not the same plant and is only minimally interchangeable. Cumin has been used traditionally to treat gas and bloating, but it is an underappreciated champion for cardiovascular health.

CUMIN SPICE BLENDS
- Fennel Dukkah Blend
- Not Necessarily Spicy Chili Blend
- Seed Blend

CUMIN RECIPES
- Dukkah Roasted Vegetables
- Red Chili Pozole
- Roasted Eggplant with Garlic Yogurt
- Sandeep's Kitchari

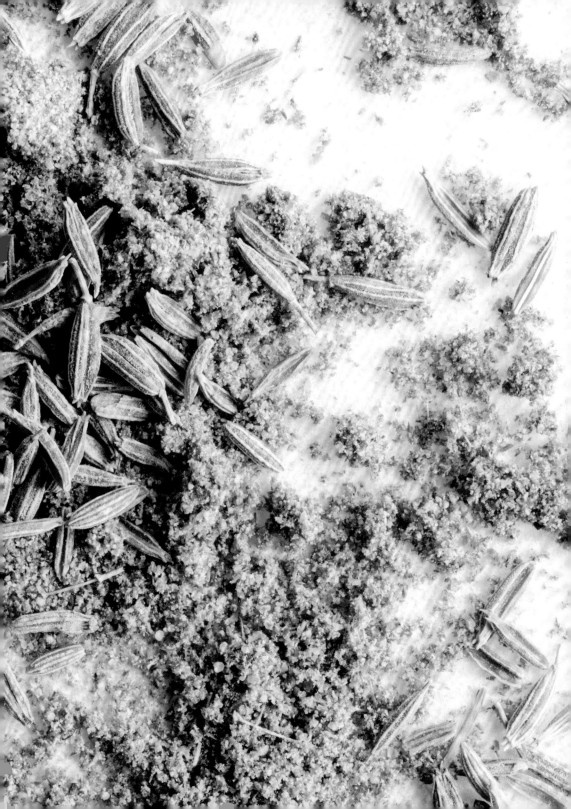

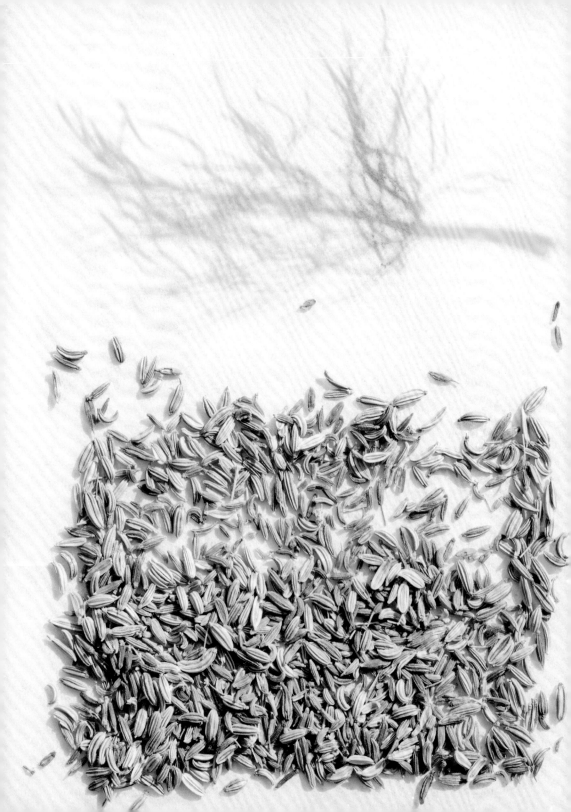

FENNEL

FOENICULUM VULGARE

Daily dose:
½ teaspoon (1.5 grams) seeds

The entire fennel plant can be used in one way or another as food and medicine. The juicy bulb is delicious grilled or shaved into a salad; and the seeds, leaves, flowers, and even pollen are potent medicinal spices. Given its licorice-like taste, fennel is a popular spice for both adults and kids. At my house, our fennel plants self-seed and return each year along the path from the front door to the driveway. When my children were babies, they'd crawl over to grab handfuls of the feathery leaves, sweet flowers, or tasty seeds. They must have thought our fennel was a magical candy bush since it presented something delicious three seasons of every year!

Fennel is wonderful medicine for all kinds of digestive upsets, but especially those impacting the lower gastrointestinal tract and causing pain, spasms, bloating, and inflammation. If your digestive tract causes you regular discomfort or pain, this may be one of the best spices choices to add to your diet.

Fennel is an easy spice to add to cooking and to make into tea. You find fennel in the French spice blend Herbs de Provence as well as in the Egyptian nut-seed-spice blend dukkah and in chai. You can also simply chew on a few seeds to help support digestion. This is common practice in India; sometimes at Indian restaurants in America you'll find a bowl of fennel seeds on the counter (often coated in candy colors) to help yourself to as you leave. Think about adding one of these small bowls of seeds to your home or office to chew on after meals.

Fennel is one of the earliest-known medicines for colic and digestive distress in infants — it can be incorporated through breast milk for a nursing child, added to food, or made into a tea from the whole seeds. There are also many traditional indications for use of fennel to support breastfeeding for lactating mothers.

FENNEL SPICE BLENDS
- Fennel Dukkah Blend
- Seed Blend
- Warming Digestive Blend

FENNEL RECIPES
- Comfy Compote
- Dukkah Roasted Vegetables
- Roasted Eggplant with Garlic Yogurt

GARLIC

ALLIUM SATIVUM

**Daily dose: 2 cloves fresh or
2 teaspoon (8.4 grams) powdered**

As an herbalist, people are always asking me what my favorite herb or spice is. Easy: garlic! Pungent garlic is a remarkable medicinal food with widely confirmed health benefits — all wrapped up in a delicate white paper case. Garlic has played a central role in herbal medicine for thousands of years. Traditionally, garlic was valued for its ability to ward off and treat infection. More recently, garlic has been shown to be an effective preventive in serious chronic health conditions, including hypertension, metabolic syndrome, and other cardiovascular conditions as well as chronic infections, immune dysregulation, and even some types of cancers.

Garlic is a powerhouse spice for the immune system and also boasts anti-inflammation and antimicrobial effects. Garlic's ability to permeate the tissues of the entire body is just one of its amazing properties. When people joke about their garlic breath sticking (stinking!) around after they eat it, it's not just their breath. The entire body absorbs garlic — skin, lungs, and blood. Here's a weird experiment to prove it: Next time you're home on a quiet Saturday night, slice open a raw clove of garlic and rub it on the soles of your feet. Within about 15 minutes, you'll be able to taste it in your mouth as it travels through your body.

If you like the taste, use garlic for daily health support. You can add it into breakfast omelets, hummus at lunch, or soups, stews, or grilling for dinner. I recommended two to three fresh cloves per day, but consuming just one per day will also have benefits.

FRESH, RAW, POWDERED, OR AGED

Using garlic in fresh bulb form is ideal. Look for bulbs with a slight purple coloring to the papery outsides; these are the most medicinal varieties. Peel the fresh cloves (there are all kinds of fun techniques to explore the best way to peel) and crack each clove by pressing it with the flat side of a knife — this allows the beneficial phytochemicals to become more potent. You can then slice or chop each clove to add to your cooking. If all that peeling sounds like too much work, you can buy pre-peeled cloves, but they are not as fresh, and some of the pungency is diminished. I would avoid buying crushed garlic in jars altogether because it lacks the medicinal punch. Instead, you can find frozen garlic or, better yet, run fresh peeled garlic through a food processor and freeze small amounts of it yourself. High-quality garlic powders and garlic granules contain a large amount of the medicinal effects of garlic in an easy-to-use form. Garlic powder, while not equivalent to the flavor of fresh garlic, is easy to use and will keep on the shelf for several months. A high-quality garlic powder can be used as a legitimate medicinal spice. I recommend two teaspoons per day if you are using garlic powder medicinally.

As an antimicrobial, garlic is best when raw. If you've eaten raw garlic before, you know it is quite strong and not very palatable to consume in large amounts. There are also some strategies for making raw garlic easier to take. When using raw garlic, it's best to coat it with something viscous. One easy method is guacamole — add raw garlic to freshly mashed avocado with lime juice and salt. You could also mix raw garlic into olive oil and spread on bread, pasta, or vegetables. Add raw garlic to peanut butter as the base of a spicy Thai peanut sauce. Or put it into honey for a sweet-savory mix. Cooked and aged garlic also have antimicrobial effects but they are significantly reduced. That doesn't mean you can't use cooked or aged garlic for antimicrobial purposes, but try to cook the garlic for as short a time as possible. Throw it in the pot at the very end of the cook time.

I love the taste of garlic, but I realize that not everyone does — and that garlic doesn't seem to love them back and can cause gastrointestinal issues. If this is the case for you, consider aged garlic extracts which are commonly available as supplements and can deliver the health effects of garlic without the flavor. Aged garlic extracts retain and concentrate some of the fresh bulb's medicinal effects, but some other beneficial constituents are lost when the garlic is aged.

FOR COLD AND INFECTION

Garlic is effective in preventing and even eliminating certain types of infection in the body. It can also be helpful on a long-term basis to benefit the cardiovascular system. You can add garlic to any of the foods you might want to eat while you are sick, including comfort foods such as chicken soup or curries. For infection, consume two to four cloves of garlic daily while you are sick.

GARLIC SPICE BLENDS

- Everyday on Everything Blend
- Green Goodness Blend
- Heart Healthy Blend
- Not Necessarily Spicy Chili Blend

GARLIC RECIPES

- Carrot-Onion-Turmeric Curry
- Eat Your Greens Pesto
- Funke's Black Soup
- Garlic Spread
- Green Goodness Dressing
- Heart Healthy Hummus
- Herby Gravy
- Medicinal Miso Soup
- Mindful Pesto
- Red Chili Pozole
- Roasted Eggplant with Garlic Yogurt
- Spicy Virgin Bloody Mary

GINGER

ZINGIBER OFFICINALE

Daily dose: 1½ teaspoons (1.5 grams) powdered or 1 teaspoon freshly grated

One taste of ginger and you'll know why this spice is believed to increase digestive fire — it's fiery! Native to Asia and most commonly used in the cuisines of China and the Indian subcontinent, ginger is hardy enough that the fresh root can be easily transported to temperate regions around the globe. I call ginger the indestructible spice because it can be dried, ground, candied, or turned into syrup or soda or soup, and it always retains its potent medicinal properties. Fresh ginger is spicy and juicy and adds a subtle aromatic flavor to cooking. In its dried form, ginger is hot, strong, and pungent. Dried ginger is used in significantly smaller amounts, typically one-tenth of the quantity of fresh by weight or volume.

Ginger is a wonderful preventive and therapeutic when colds and flus come around. Ginger can also be used daily for long-term immune support, desirable for those with immune imbalances. It's also wonderful for infectious illnesses with digestive implications due to its ability to calm nausea and soothe irritated digestive mucosa. Traditionally used to warm up the body and support diaphoresis (sweating) and the natural fever response, the use of a hot bath with a hot cup of ginger tea is a timeless method of supporting the body during an acute infectious illness. A favorite preparation is Hot Ginger Lemonade (page 152) made with fresh ginger. When family gathers in the winter months and colds readily spread around, this is something I like to keep on the stove ready for the young and old to dip a ladle into and fill a mug to keep us well.

BOOST THE BRAIN

Not commonly used for its effects on cognition, ginger is worth considering based on a few pieces of recent research. In clinical trials, people who took 400 mg or 800 mg of ginger (administered as an alcohol extract dried into powder) every day for two months showed significant improvement in cognitive assessments, including auditory and visual stimuli with verbal, pictorial, numerical, and spatial components; working memory; recognition; and reaction time. These are relatively high doses of ginger for culinary use, so you could consider food preparations that allow for an easy way to consume a lot of ginger. The research and safety data on ginger is extensive and points to regular dietary use.

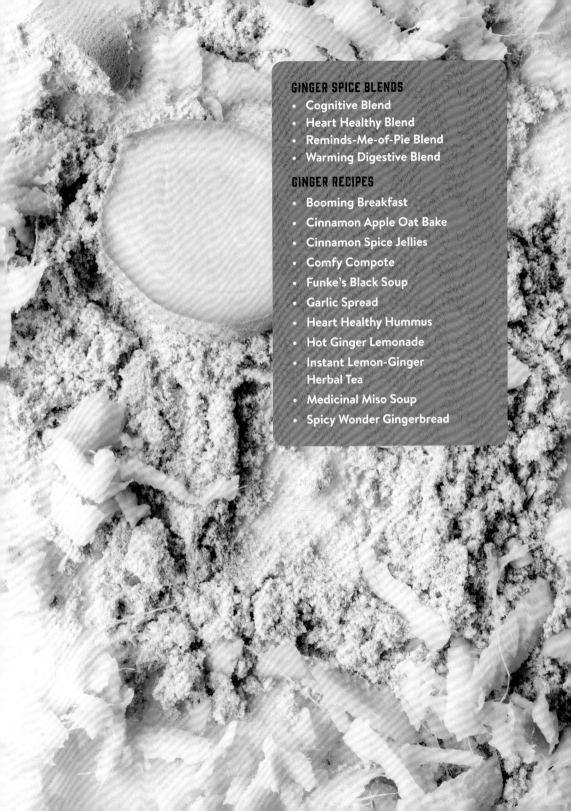

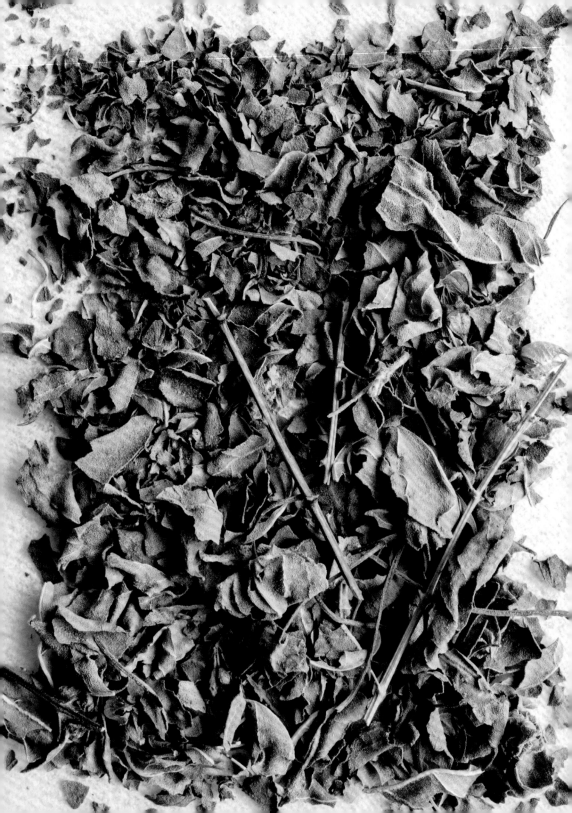

HOLY BASIL

OCIMUM SANCTUM

Daily dose:
2 teaspoons (1.6 grams) cut and sifted

Holy basil, also known as tulsi, has been used traditionally for medicinal purposes in India for centuries. Recent research has shown that while all types of basil have significant antioxidant and anti-inflammatory properties, holy basil is the most potent. You may want to try swapping out sweet basil for holy basil in your cooking. If you find that holy basil tastes too medicinal or intense, you can always use half sweet and half holy in a dish.

You can often find holy basil at Asian grocery stores alongside Thai basil. If you can't find it fresh, you can opt for dried. It's also very easy to grow. Holy basil is more drought-tolerant and hardier than sweet basil, and grows well in a small pot even on a city windowsill.

Used in cuisines around the world from Latin America to Asia to Europe and India, basil's captivating flavor pairs well with tomato, balsamic vinegar, and chili pepper. The delicate leaf of the plant is best used freshly picked, as it tends to wilt and brown rather quickly, but basil can also be used mashed, ground, dried, or frozen. Many of us are familiar with Italian basil, or sweet basil. But there are a variety of different basils, all in the mint family, including lemon basil, Thai basil, and holy basil. While they share a semi-sweet aromatic taste, some are more pungent than others, and some even have a licorice-like taste.

HOLY BASIL SPICE BLENDS
- Cognitive Blend
- Everyday on Everything Blend
- Green Goodness Blend
- Heart Healthy Blend

HOLY BASIL RECIPES
- Booming Breakfast
- Eat Your Greens Pesto
- Garlic Spread
- Green Goodness Dressing
- Heart Healthy Hummus
- Herby Gravy
- Medicinal Miso Soup
- Mindful Pesto
- Spicy Virgin Bloody Mary

LAVENDER

LAVANDULA ANGUSTIFOLIA

Daily dose:
1 teaspoon (1 gram) dried flowers

Lavender is known and loved in the world of essential oils and is often used to support a healthy nervous system. The plant is used less frequently as a spice in food but it is beneficial. You'll find it in the French spice blend Herbs de Provence, which includes thyme, marjoram, summer savory, rosemary, oregano, basil, sage, and lavender.

Lavender lends a floral taste to foods and works well when blended with rosemary and used in small amounts on savory meat and vegetable dishes. The flowers can quickly overpower but can lend a balance in small amounts to strong-tasting foods such as wild game, pungent cheeses, or strongly flavored herb and spice blends. While the leaves look similar to many other aromatic leaves used in Mediterranean cooking, they have a strong bitter element and are best avoided in food. Some people do have an aversion to lavender in food and experience it as soapy in flavor. Used in the right amount, it can be a great celebratory addition to baked sweets. Add ground lavender flowers to sugar to create a lavender sugar and make lavender lemonade or lavender cookies.

LAVENDER SPICE BLEND
- Cognitive Blend

LAVENDER RECIPE
- Blooming Breakfast

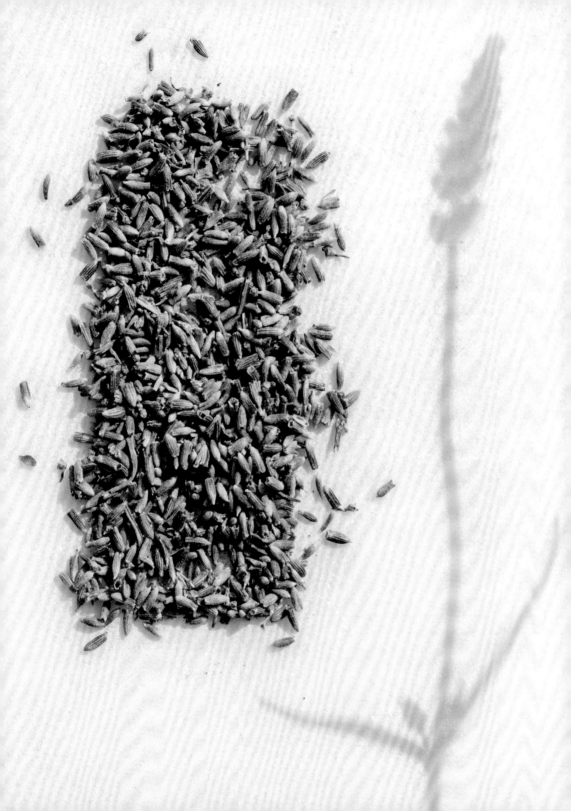

MINT'S AROMATICS AND TANNINS

There are two prominent constituent groups in mint: aromatics and tannins. The aromatics are the "minty" aspects of the plant; these are what we want to extract for medicinal use. The tannins are astringents, which can be used to tighten and tone mucous membranes, but they aren't generally desirable in mint preparations in more than a small amount. Tannins might make your mouth feel tight or dry, such as with strong black tea or dry wine. So, we try to use extractions that pull out the aromatics while leaving behind the tannins.

Here's a fun experiment that demonstrates the delicate volatile nature of mint: prepare dried mint three different ways and taste to compare. For the first preparation, soak dried mint (or a mint tea bag) in room temperature water overnight without exposing it to heat. This will bring out the volatile oils without the tannins. In a second preparation, boil dried mint (or a mint tea bag) for 15 minutes. The room will smell great, but when you let the tea cool you'll find it has almost no minty flavor left. Finally, make an infusion by pouring boiling water over dried mint (or tea bag) and let it sit for just one minute with a cover over it. This will retain the volatile oils best while minimizing the tannins.

MINT

MENTHA SPP.

**Daily dose:
1 tablespoon (3.3 grams) cut and sifted**

Mint is used extensively in dishes around the globe — chopped fresh and added to salads or noodles or to fresh rice paper rolls, as in Vietnamese cuisine. Fresh mint is also popular in cocktails, like the mojito. It makes a prominent appearance in British cuisine in mint sauce used as an accompaniment to meat dishes. Mint is easy to grow — although, be careful, it will take over your garden! Best to grow it in a pot or a dedicated garden bed. When preparing mint for cooking, it's important to note that high or prolonged heat can destroy the delicate volatile oils and beneficial astringent tannins that give mint its medicinal properties. I advise using fresh, uncooked mint whenever possible. If using dried mint, keep it at low heat, or add it to the dish after cooking.

When we think of mint, we are most commonly thinking of the aromatic oils of peppermint, (*Mentha piperita*) or that of its close relative, spearmint. There are many mints in the genus, and only some of them are used in culinary applications. In general, you can use peppermint or spearmint in any recipe that calls for mint, but other mints cannot always be used in place of these two.

Mint is palatable and gentle. Mint tea is a common treatment for an upset stomach. The tea can be made with dried or fresh mint leaves, and a variety of different types of mint might be used — peppermint, spearmint, pineapple mint, or chocolate mint. Mint has been shown to be helpful for nearly all types of gastrointestinal upsets, from gallbladder discomfort to pregnancy nausea to dyspepsia and even inflammatory bowel disease. For any of these conditions, using mint can help regulate gastric tone and spasms.

MINT SPICE BLENDS
- Cognitive Blend
- Mint and Chile Blend

MINT RECIPES
- Booming Breakfast
- Minty Yogurt Spread

MUSTARD

BRASSICA NIGRA

Daily dose:
½ teaspoon (1.3 grams) powdered

Mustard often gets shelved in the condiment category and is underemployed as a spice in itself. This tiny seed, native to North Africa, is more closely related to common leafy *Brassica* vegetables such as collards, kale, broccoli, and arugula than it is to other spices — except horseradish, which is a close relative.

When we talk about mustard seed we are generally referring to *Brassica nigra*, though there are others, such as brown Indian mustard (*Brassica juncea*) and white or yellow mustard seeds (*Brassica hirta* and *Brassica alba*). Mustard's pungency might be more flexible than you realize, and once you start playing with the dried and ground seeds, you'll find yourself adding it to more and more dishes.

Mustard seed (also known as black mustard seed) can be consumed as a whole dried seed, or the seed can be powdered (typically with the outer coating removed). It can also be prepared as a spreadable sauce we are all familiar with. Prepared mustard spreads were originally made by grinding yellow or Dijon mustard seeds and adding vinegar. The preparation hasn't changed much over time other than the addition of salt, fancy vinegar, or sometimes turmeric. It's a simple, affordable, tasty, and accessible spice preparation that people use every day without knowing about its medicinal benefits.

PUNGENT MEDICINE

The flavor of dried mustard seeds alone is relatively mild, but the addition of water causes an enzymatic release of the pungent mustard oil, and it can be spicy! Indian cuisine often uses whole mustard seeds, adding them to hot oil and letting them pop and spread flavor throughout the oil and the dish. The pungent spice of mustard seed begins to fade and become milder after cooking them for about 15 minutes. Adding hot water or acid such as vinegar or lemon juice to a dish will also tame the heat. Mustard is delicious in curries, and you might be surprised that you can even use it in sweets alongside other pungent herbs like ginger. A favorite of mine is the Spicy Wonder Gingerbread (see page 123) which features both of these tasty medicinal spices.

Medicinally, mustard plays an important role in many cultures. It is used to generate heat and warmth. Hot mustard baths, for example, are a common treatment for cold or a flu, especially when there is respiratory impairment. Mustard plasters, where dried mustard powder is mixed with flour and water and used as a poultice, have been used for millennia for infections and congestion of the respiratory system. Mustard plasters are made by combining dried mustard powder with flour at a 1-to-3 ratio and mixing with water to form a thick spread. The spread is put on a thin cloth and draped across the patient's back and chest for 15 minutes.

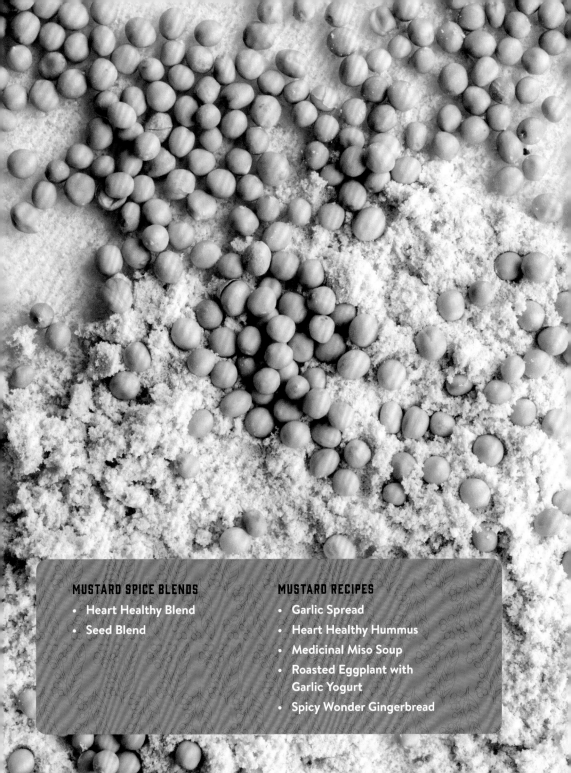

MUSTARD SPICE BLENDS

- Heart Healthy Blend
- Seed Blend

MUSTARD RECIPES

- Garlic Spread
- Heart Healthy Hummus
- Medicinal Miso Soup
- Roasted Eggplant with Garlic Yogurt
- Spicy Wonder Gingerbread

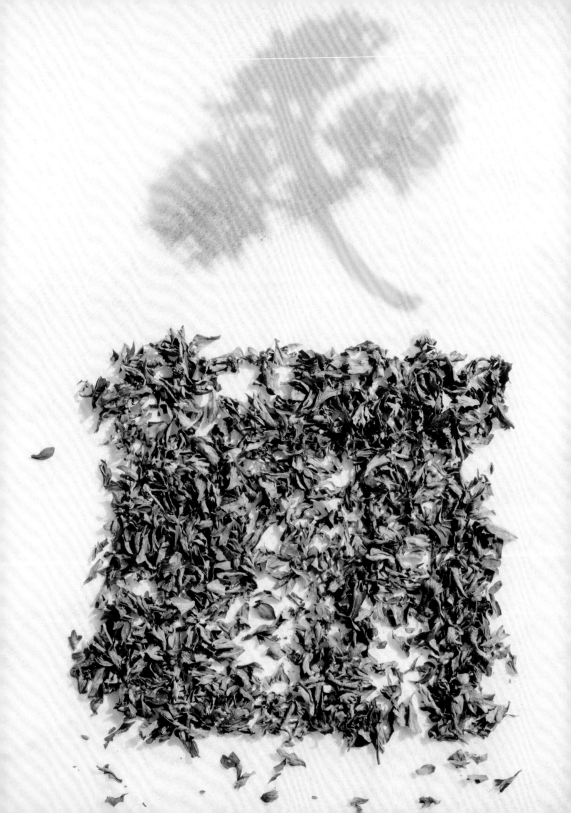

PARSLEY

PETROSELINUM CRISPUM

Daily dose: 1 tablespoon (2.3 grams) chopped fresh or cut and sifted

For many years, parsley was simply a garnish on our plates (this now seems to have gone out of fashion). It's a common item at grocery stores in fresh bunches, curly or flat, which gives me hope that there are many admirers of this fresh medicinal herb.

Parsley is best used fresh, which is readily available and inexpensive. Freshly chopped parsley can be added to all sorts of savory dishes. You can throw it into almost anything that includes other Mediterranean spices, like basil, thyme, oregano, or rosemary. It is a prominent ingredient in Middle Eastern dishes such as tabbouleh, a salad of parsley, bulgur wheat, mint, tomato, and olive oil. And check out the Parsley Pesto recipe (page 149) to get your daily dose in a delicious spread made with lemons and pistachios. Feel free to use parsley in large amounts; its mild green flavor makes it easy to pick up a bunch and start experimenting.

If you can't get fresh parsley you can use dried, but it has a very short shelf life and can be relatively expensive compared to fresh. If you use dried parsley, try to buy small amounts and use it up quickly. You can tell that dried parsley is no longer fresh when it loses its vibrant green color and turns pale yellow or brown. To use parsley medicinally on a regular basis, you'll want to consume at least a tablespoon of finely chopped fresh or dried parsley daily.

PARSLEY SPICE BLEND
• Green Goodness Blend

PARSLEY RECIPES
• Green Goodness Dressing
• Parsley Pesto

ROSEMARY

ROSEMARINUS OFFICINALIS

Daily dose:
½ teaspoon (1 gram) cut and sifted

The strong, resinous needles of this Mediterranean shrub are delicious and evoke the sun-soaked coast of the hot and dry lands where they originate. Rosemary leaves have such a strong antioxidant capacity they are used to preserve foods, such as delicate oils, from becoming rancid. These same antioxidant compounds can also help "preserve" some of your cognitive processes and capabilities.

The beneficial medicinal effects of rosemary have been known for a long time; Shakespeare informs us in *Hamlet* that rosemary is for remembrance. This delicious medicinal plant can be grown easily in a pot outdoors during the summer or as a perennial in warmer regions, and if you have a green thumb you might be able to keep it happy indoors in a sunny window.

Using the fresh needles is far superior to using dried rosemary. Fresh rosemary needles can be chopped finely and added into food for maximum flavor and absorption; dried rosemary, on the other hand, can be a bit tough to chew. If you can't get fresh rosemary, dried is fine if you grind it yourself prior to using it. Powdered rosemary loses the delicious oils quickly and doesn't have wonderful flavor.

ROSEMARY SPICE BLENDS

- Cognitive Blend
- Everyday on Everything Blend
- Heart Healthy Blend

ROSEMARY RECIPES

- Booming Breakfast
- Heart Healthy Hummus
- Herby Gravy
- Mindful Pesto
- Spicy Virgin Bloody Mary

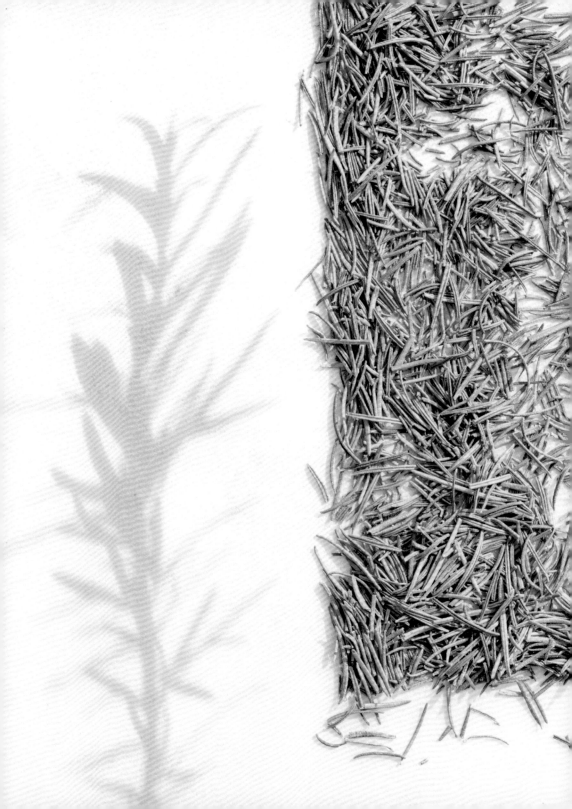

SAGE

SALVIA OFFICINALIS

Daily dose:
½ teaspoon (0.5 grams) cut and sifted

This common kitchen herb is easy to grow in the garden and is also perfectly good when used dried. Sage has a strong flavor and is typically used in small amounts in cooking. Often found in butter-based sauces of French and Italian cooking, sage is good in most savory Mediterranean dishes alongside rosemary, thyme, or oregano. Its strong flavor can take some getting used to if you aren't accustomed to it, but its unique medicinal actions make it a worthy addition to your apothecary.

To use sage medicinally, I recommend at least ½ teaspoon of dried herb per day. Some conditions may call for more, but this is a good amount to start with as you explore ways to integrate the strong flavor into your diet. It's also a perfect spice to use in fresh form and is easy to grow in many climates. To use it fresh, add 3 to 4 leaves to a recipe.

SAGE SPICE BLEND
- Everyday on Everything Blend

SAGE RECIPES
- Herby Gravy
- Spicy Virgin Bloody Mary

THYME

THYMUS VULGARIS

Daily dose:
1½ teaspoons (1.3 grams) powdered

Thyme thrives in a desert environment and is protected by the potent aromatic oils in its leaves. These oils, which the plant uses to ward off predators and disease, can also be used by our bodies for antimicrobial protection and defense.

The flavor of this tiny leaf is anything but tiny. It is employed in many cuisines around the world, most notably in Mediterranean cuisines and some cuisines of the Caribbean, such as Jamaican. It can be added to most savory dishes and makes good company with sage and rosemary. Thyme can be cooked for a long period of time and still retain its flavor, although it may be reduced in pungency. It's also one of the easiest plants to grow if you have plenty of sunshine. You can plant it in a pot or in the ground, and it doesn't need much to stay happy.

Thyme can be eaten in large doses safely and has traditionally been used to treat respiratory infections. One of my favorite uses for thyme is as a respiratory steam or a gargle for a sore throat. For the sore throat gargle, make a simple tea or infusion of thyme and allow it to cool, then add a pinch of salt. Gargle with the mixture several times per day.

THYME SPICE BLEND
- Cognitive Blend

THYME RECIPE
- Blooming Breakfast

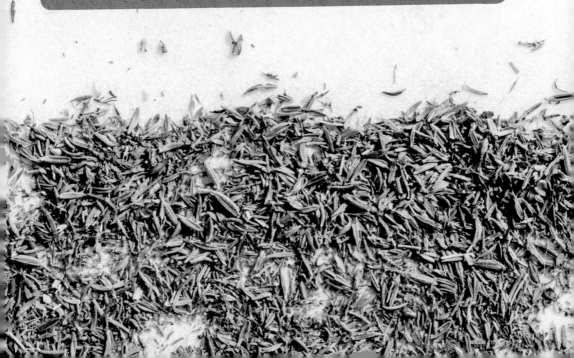

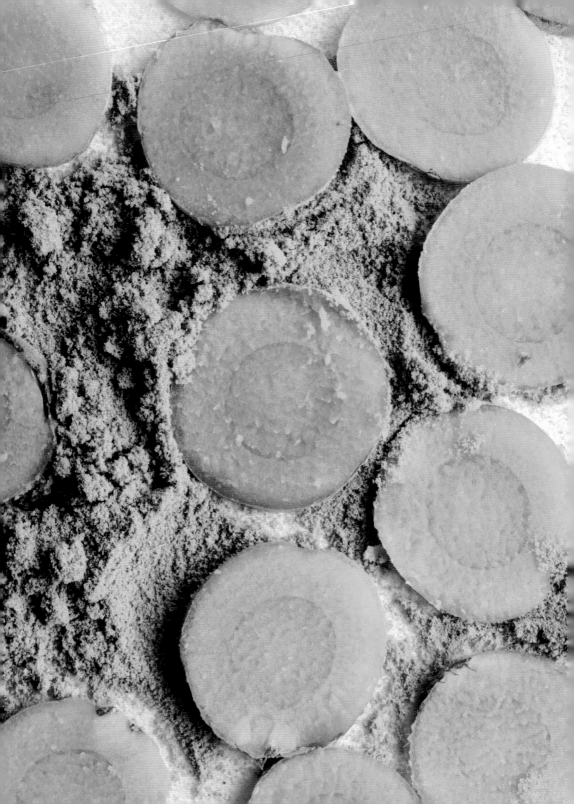

TURMERIC

CURCUMA LONGA

Daily dose:
½ teaspoon (1.7 grams) powdered

Turmeric offers protection from inflammation anywhere in the body, making it an excellent medicinal spice for working with conditions of the bones, skin, and joints. As chronic problems of the heart tend to center around inflammation, turmeric is also a natural choice to address common concerns surrounding diseases of the heart.

Turmeric has been used as a medicinal plant for centuries in India and China. Its numerous benefits seem to derive from the chemical constituents found in curcumin, a chemical compound that makes up about 2 to 5 percent of the chemical composition of this rhizome. Many commercial supplement products on the market focus solely or mainly on this isolated constituent despite the plethora of compounds present in the rhizome. One study has also shown that curcumin is not the only medicinally active constituent in turmeric. Many constituents have been shown to have medicinal actions independent of curcumin. Turmeric in its whole form has been found to include the following beneficial properties: anti-inflammatory, anti-microbial, antioxidant, antidepressant, anticancer, antimutagenic, radioprotective, hepatoprotective, neuroprotective, antidiabetic, wound-healing, and anti-aging.

It may sound like a cure-all, but there are so many ways to add this vibrant spice to your food, it's worth throwing a half-teaspoon into your cooking each day. From complex Indian curries to sweet golden milk, turmeric offers a bright way to stave off inflammation throughout the whole body. Have a look at the recipes for Heart Synergy Fudge (page 139), Hot Ginger Lemonade (page 152), and Medicinal Miso Soup (page 147) for excellent ways to get your daily dose of turmeric.

TURMERIC SPICE BLENDS

- Cognitive Blend
- Everyday on Everything Blend
- Fennel Dukkah Blend
- Green Goodness Blend
- Heart Healthy Blend
- Peppery Synergy Blend
- Warming Digestive Blend

TURMERIC RECIPES

- Booming Breakfast
- Carrot-Onion-Turmeric Curry
- Comfy Compote
- Dukkah Roasted Vegetables
- Garlic Spread
- Green Goodness Dressing
- Heart Healthy Hummus
- Heart Synergy Fudge
- Herby Gravy
- Instant Lemon-Ginger Herbal Tea
- Medicinal Miso Soup
- Sandeep's Kitchari
- Spicy Virgin Bloody Mary

SPICES AROUND THE GLOBE: ZANZIBAR

THE ISLAND OF ZANZIBAR lies off the coast of Tanzania in eastern Africa, and its soil and climate are ideal for growing tropical spices. I visited the Tangawizi Spice Farm in central Zanzibar where they grow turmeric, ginger, vanilla, lemongrass, nutmeg, mace, black pepper, cloves, cinnamon, and cardamom. The educational farm welcomes visitors into the forest to see how spices grow in the wild, helping visitors gain an understanding of the biodiversity and ecosystem where spices thrive. The flowers, fruits, and scents under the thick canopy are all part of the vivid wonder of this tropical forest. There is something magical about pulling bark straight from the cinnamon tree, nibbling a flower bud and discovering the taste of cloves, and sniffing a vanilla orchid flower!

I was curious to know if Tanzanians use the same parts of the plant that we do for spices or, with the whole plant at their disposal, they use other parts for food and medicine. One of the farmers at Tangawizi talked with me about some of the common uses of these spices, starting with one of my favorites.

Cinnamon is traditionally used for overall health as well as for weight loss, high blood pressure, and diabetes. To prepare it, they typically boil the dried bark for five minutes and drink it as a tea, one cup per day. Interestingly, this aligns with best practices shown in contemporary research. In addition to making use of the bark, they also use the aromatic roots as a vapor rub or massage oil for treating colds and flu.

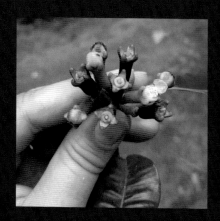

Clove buds (*Syzygium aromaticum*) at the Tangawizi Spice Farm in Zanzibar.

Cloves are abundant in Zanzibar. They are used to treat toothache — clove powder is applied directly to the toothbrush. To support bone health, cloves are added to food as a spice. And for stomach problems, clove buds are chewed and swallowed with water.

Turmeric is focused on brain health. To use it, the powdered rhizome is mixed with egg yolks or taken in milk; these methods provide the lipids that make the spice bioavailable. Turmeric is also helpful for stomach ulcers; turmeric powder is combined with egg yolk, coconut milk, and honey, and two teaspoons are taken two times per day for two months. They also use turmeric topically for skin conditions by mixing the powder with water and lemon juice, applying it to the skin, and letting it rest for 30 to 45 minutes before washing.

Ginger is used to support the immune system and to treat coughs, colds, and stomach issues. To prepare ginger, it is freshly juiced and mixed with turmeric powder and lemon juice.

Meeting these spices up close made them come alive for me in ways that the dried versions I find back home cannot. Now, every time I smell cloves, I am transported to Zanzibar to that thriving forest full of abundance.

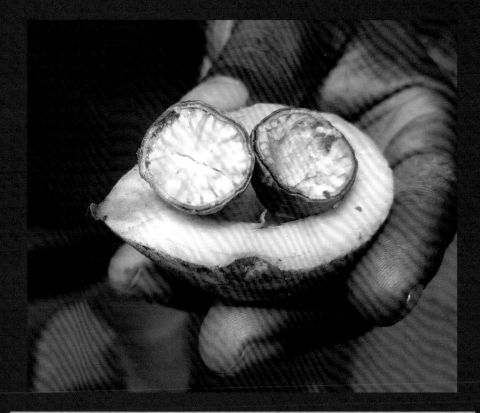

The fresh fruit and seed of *Myristica fragrans* at Tangawizi Spice Farm in Zanzibar, from which both nutmeg (from the seed) and mace (from the seed covering) are used as spices

MEDICINAL USE AND DOSAGE

MEDICINAL SPICE	BOTANICAL NAME	PART USED	USE FRESH	USE DRY	USE POWDER
BLACK PEPPER	Piper nigrum	FRUIT		X	X
CALENDULA	Calendula officialis	PETALS	X	X	
CARDAMON	Ellettaria cardamomum	SEED POD		X	X
CELERY SEED	Apium graveloens	SEED		X	X
CHILES	Capsicum spp.	FRUIT	X	X	X
CINNAMON	Cinnamomum verum	BARK		X	X
CUMIN	Cuminum cyminum	SEED		X	X
FENNEL	Foeniculum vulgare	SEED		X	X
GARLIC	Allium sativum	BULB	X	X	X
GINGER	Zingiber officinale	RHIZOME	X	X	X
HOLY BASIL	Ocimum sanctum	LEAF	X	X	
LAVENDER	Lavandula angustifolia	FLOWER		X	
MINT	Mentha piperita, M. spp	LEAF	X	X	
MUSTARD	Brassica nigra	SEED		X	X
PARSLEY	Petroselinum crispum	LEAF	X	X	
ROSEMARY	Rosmarinus officinalis	LEAF	X	X	
SAGE	Salvia officinalis	LEAF	X	X	
THYME	Thymus vulgaris	LEAF	X	X	
TURMERIC	Curcuma longa	RHIZOME	X	X	X

KEY **c/s:** cut and sifted **pwd:** powdered

USE WHOLE OR C/S	DAILY DOSE	DAILY DOSE IN GRAMS
	¼ tsp pwd	1
X	2 tsp fresh	0.5–1
X	¼ tsp pwd	0.8
X	¼ tsp seed	1.5
	sprinkle	0.25–0.5
	¼ tsp pwd	1–2
X	¼ tsp pwd or seed	1–2
X	½ tsp seed	1–2
X	2 cloves fresh or 1 tsp pwd	2–3
X	½ tsp pwd	1–2
X	2 tsp c/s	1.6
X	2 tsp	1
X	1 tbsp c/s	3.3
X	½ tsp	1.3
X	1 tbsp fresh or c/s	2.3
X	½ tsp c/s	0.5
X	½ tsp c/s	0.5
X	½ tsp	1
	½ tsp	1.7

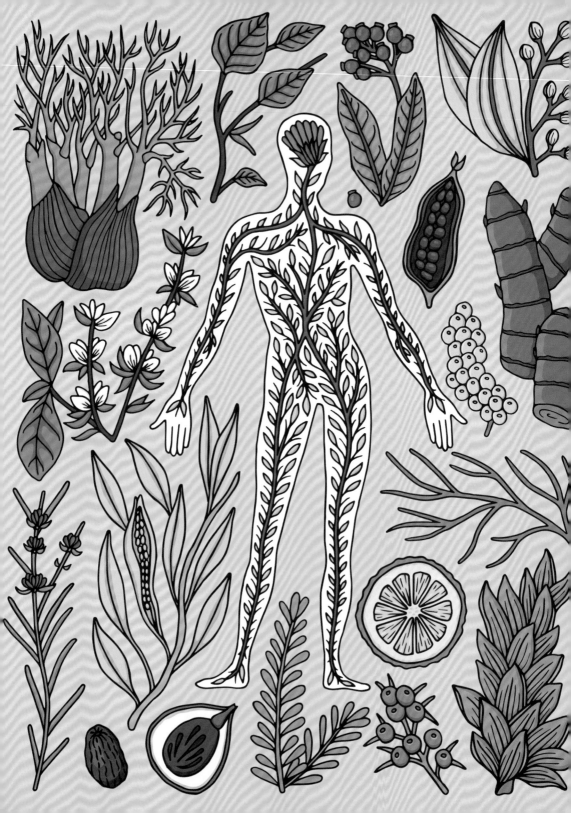

CHAPTER 4

Using Spices to Support Health Goals

Spices can offer targeted support for specific health goals and functions of the body. Whether you've been diagnosed with hypertension, want to reduce inflammation in your knees, or address digestive issues or lung problems, the benefits of filling your diet with aromatic spices is supported by scientific evidence. The clinical studies on the use of spices to support the seven health goals in this chapter are all listed in the bibliography.

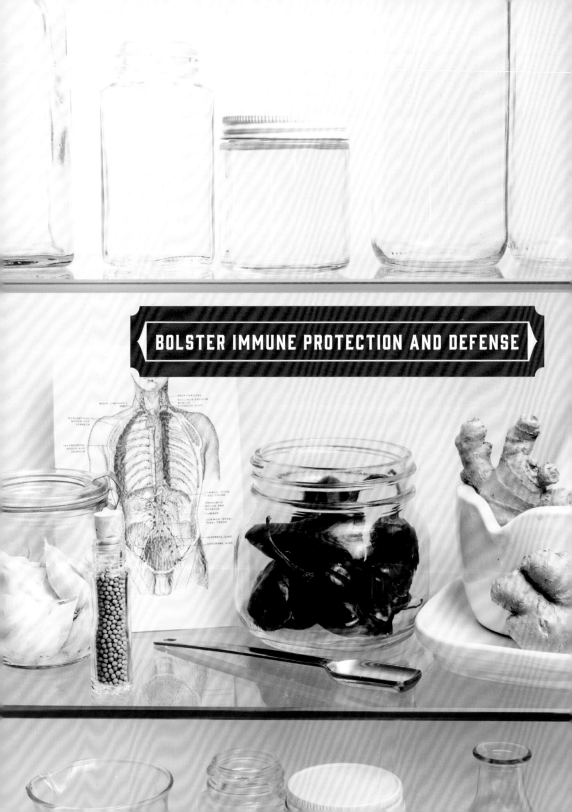

BOLSTER IMMUNE PROTECTION AND DEFENSE

OUR BODIES ARE, and exist within, ecosystems. We interact constantly with other organisms that both surround us and live inside us. Protection from harmful organisms or viruses is a never-ending negotiation, and we are well-equipped for the task with our complex and nimble immune systems. That doesn't mean we never succumb to infections, as we are all too aware. Supporting the body to have greater defenses, as well as its ability to fight back when it does get sick, are arenas where spices can help. All spices are anti-inflammatory in one way or another, and this aspect alone can support our body and its defenses. There are also numerous spices that are potent antimicrobials. Yet other herbs and spices are more gentle and can be used in cases of immune imbalances or with a more sensitive system.

When you're looking to support protection and defense during an infection, the concept of "terrain" is central, meaning the general ecosystem of your body and how hospitable it is to pathogenic organisms. For example, the consumption of a lot of sweets can create a more favorable environment for certain types of bacteria, viruses, and fungi, which makes infection more likely when you are otherwise compromised or exposed. When you eat aromatic spices they penetrate throughout much of your tissues. Specifically, chile, garlic, ginger, and mustard create a less conducive environment for certain types of infectious pathogens. They warm up the body, reduce inflammation, increase circulation, and make the body a less hospitable place for pathogens to thrive, replicate, and spread.

When we talk about changing the terrain of the body, the idea is to increase overall aromatic and spiced food consumption in order to increase the body's ability to deal with pathogens or infection. When a cold or virus is going around in your community, the simple measure of consuming more spices can be helpful. And in cases of chronic infection, it can be a good step in a treatment strategy to move back to health.

In sufficient quantity, ginger, garlic, chili, and mustard can play a role in shifting terrain. They can be used fresh or powdered, singularly or as a blend, and can be used in smaller, regular doses or in larger, more concentrated doses in acute situations. You might use mustard and garlic in your food once a day to support overall health during the change of seasons when you're prone to getting sick. And if you find yourself coming down with something and want to rally your defenses, you could prepare a larger amount of it in the recipe for Medicinal Miso Soup (see page 145). While all of these spices are safe in large doses, it's important to know how your body handles spicy or pungent foods and to stay within your comfort zone.

GARLIC *Allium sativum*

Garlic has a well-docmented history of use for immune function, and for its antibacterial and antimicrobial properties. It has a broad antibiotic spectrum against both gram-positive and gram-negative bacteria and has been proven to inhibit *Aerobacter, Aeromonas, Bacillus, Citrella, Citrobacter, Clostridium, Enterobacter, Escherichia, Klebsiella, Lactobacillus, Leuconostoc, Micrococcus,*

Mycobacterium, Proteus, Providencia, Pseudomonas, Salmonella, Serratia, Shigella, Staphylococcus, Streptococcus, and *Vibrio* as well as *Helicobacter pylori.* It has been shown to be synergistic with some pharmaceutical antibiotics and not be prone to antibiotic resistance by pathogens.

One study examined the effect of garlic on the body's ability to fight the common cold. Participants took a garlic supplement for a 12-week period during the winter months and kept a daily record of their symptoms. During this period the garlic group had just 37 percent of the colds compared to those of the control group. Furthermore, the placebo group was more likely to get more than one cold per season compared to the garlic group.

Garlic receives high marks for immunomodulation and anti-inflammatory effects. These aspects of garlic have been proposed as promising candidates for maintaining the homeostasis of the immune system. The anti-inflammatory effects of garlic compounds may contribute to the treatment and prevention of pathologies such as obesity, metabolic syndrome, cardiovascular disease, gastric ulcer, and even cancer. Several studies have examined garlic's ability to prevent the associated harm from *Helicobacter pylori* infection, a leading cause of gastric cancer.

CHILE *Capsicum* spp.

Chile peppers of all types are rich in antioxidant and anti-inflammatory benefits. Peppers of the *Capsicum annuum* species have been shown to have both antibacterial and antifungal properties against *Bacillus subtilis, Staphylococcus aureus, Staphylococcus epidermidis, Escherichia coli,* and *Candida albicans.*

GINGER *Zingiber officinale*

Ginger and its constituents have been widely researched and have been found to have antioxidant, anti-inflammatory, anti-nausea, and antimutagenic properties. It has been shown to suppress the growth and induce cell death of a variety of types of cancer. A review of clinical studies on ginger's protective role in gastrointestinal disorders found that ginger has potential chemopreventive effects against colorectal cancer. In one study, the anti-inflammatory effects of ginger were apparent, lowering COX-1 protein expression (an inflammatory marker) in those with increased risk for colorectal cancer but not in those at normal risk.

MUSTARD *Brassica nigra*

Mustard is an ideal medicine for bronchial infections of the damp and stagnant type. It is helpful when a strong expectorant is needed or when there is lingering phlegm in the respiratory system. Its medicinal benefits over the long term are similar to that of the brassicas, which are known to be powerfully anti-inflammatory and anti-cancer, perhaps even more concentrated. Some of our understanding of the medicinal benefits of mustard seed is gleaned from our knowledge of its relatives in the Brassica family. Mustard seed, like its cousins, contains glucosinolates, known for anti-inflammatory and anti-cancer actions. Moreover, mustard seed also contains enzymes that break down glucosinolates to release the even more powerfully medicinal isothiocyanates. These isothiocyanates are powerful modulators of the expression and activity of enzymes that are involved in the metabolism and elimination of a variety of carcinogens from the body.

The research on mustard may surprise you. One clinical trial studied the effects of four spices on diet-induced thermogenesis (DIT), an increase in energy expenditure over metabolic rate caused by food, which could be an aid to weight loss. Mustard, ginger, horseradish, and black pepper were tested on subjects who fasted with no intake of alcohol, caffeine, or hot spices for the previous 24 hours and no physical exercise in the previous 48 hours. A number of measures were noted, including weight, body mass composition, respiration, and urine and blood samples. The subjects were then given a meal of bread, ham, scrambled eggs, butter, fruit, beets, fruit juice, and water that included about 14 grams of one of the four spices. After the subjects ate the meal, measurements for energy balance and thermogenic effect were taken for four hours following. Only mustard showed an improvement over placebo. Although the increase was slight, it suggests that regular consumption of mustard has the potential to increase DIT and thereby be an adjunct to maintaining optimal weight.

A related clinical trial found a positive effect of mustard on both satiety and glycemic response. Healthy participants ate a meal of potato and leek soup — with or without the addition of 5 grams of yellow mustard bran. Satiety and capillary blood glucose were measured at intervals for two hours following the meal. Blood glucose levels were significantly lower with the addition of the mustard.

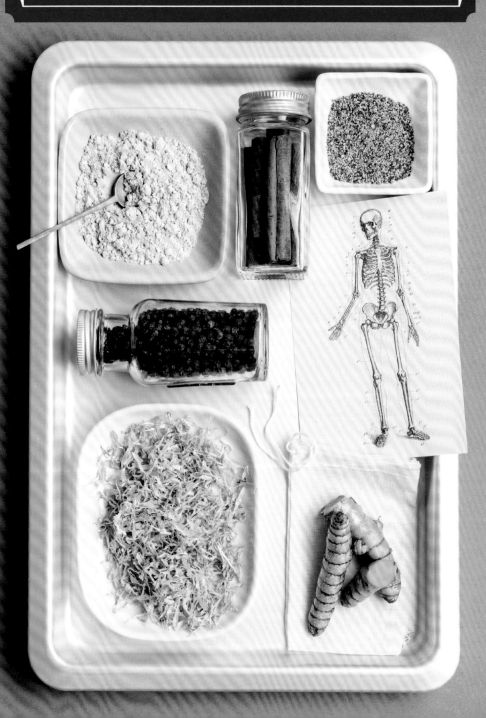

OUR SKIN IS the organ that interacts most with the world. A dynamic and responsive organ, it contends with all kinds of impacts and intrusions. It can also reflect what is going on internally, including hormonal changes and liver function. We might notice skin changes in people with declining or challenged liver function as well as in those who are exposed to certain types of toxins. In these situations, you'll want to use spices that are both internally effective as well as topically helpful.

Black pepper, calendula, cinnamon, ginger, and turmeric can all be used therapeutically on a daily basis for the internal and external environment affecting skin health. The spicy punch of these plants can also help improve circulation and mobilization in the connective tissues of the body.

Calendula, turmeric, and ginger are all great spices to consider in support of your bones, joints, and skin. Degenerative joint diseases such as arthritis are prevalent globally, and the research around the use of spices as therapeutics is compelling for both ginger and turmeric.

Unlike conventional medications, which are taken after symptoms begin, the use of these spices can be life-long and preventive. Using ginger in conjunction with turmeric has a long history of use in supporting joint health, both topically and internally. Traditional application of ginger poultices, hot ginger compresses, and ginger-infused baths are used to treat painful joints. Ginger is a wonderful preventive against joint disease and boosts health by aiding the reduction of pain and swelling. It is accessible and affordable in fresh form, which makes it a superior choice as a medicine.

CINNAMON *Cinnamomum* spp.

Cinnamon is useful in addressing inflammation in skin, bones, or joints. It has a beneficial impact on hypertension and managing blood sugar, both of which are linked to chronic inflammation. Cinnamon has also been shown to have positive effects on treating rheumatoid arthritis. A group of patients who received a daily dose of 500 mg of cinnamon for eight weeks (2 grams total) showed significantly lower C-reactive protein, tumor necrosis factor alpha, and diastolic blood pressure. These results indicate reduced inflammation as well as an improvement in swollen and tender joints in the body.

TURMERIC *Curcuma longa*

Turmeric has been shown to benefit skin disorders, including psoriasis. In one trial, a topical skin treatment containing turmeric showed significant improvement over the pharmaceutical cream calcipotriol as well as was the control group. It was also was discovered to decrease pro-inflammatory cytokines in human keratinocytes, thereby reducing keratinocyte hyperproliferation found in psoriasis. The same study found that wound healing was enhanced by curcumin's actions as an anti-inflammatory agent and a reactive oxygen species (ROS) scavenger. Curcumin has also been shown to enhance cell proliferation; reverse oxidative damage to skin cells, fibroblasts, and keratinocytes; and facilitate faster healing of the epidermis.

GINGER *Zingiber officinale*

Ginger is touted for its analgesic and anti-inflammatory effects. One trial found that daily consumption of ginger, raw or cooked, significantly reduced the pain of exercise-induced muscle injury within 24 hours. In a two-phase trial, muscle injury was induced in participants through repetitive exercise of the elbow flexor muscles, and participants were randomly and blindly assigned a daily dose of 2 grams ginger or placebo for 11 days. In the first phase, raw ginger was studied and was found to have a 25-percent reduction in muscle pain 24 hours after exercise. In the second phase, heat-treated ginger was studied and had a 23-percent reduction in pain. A trial group that received 4 grams of ginger for five days had lower post-exercise pain scales as well as lower blood markers (creatine kinase) for muscle damage.

In a study looking at ginger in patients with knee osteoarthritis, 120 patients were randomly assigned to receive 500 mg of ginger powder or placebo daily for three months. This small, food-like dose decreased a number of inflammatory factors in the patients as compared to the placebo.

CALENDULA *Calendula officinalis*

Calendula has long been used as a healing agent for the skin and soft tissues and has traditionally been applied topically. Its medicinal effects can be significant in serious situations, such as radiation burns (related to cancer treatment) and gastric ulcers. One study compared the use of calendula against a saline solution dressing for the topical treatment of leg ulcers, measured by reepithelialization. Patients who were given an application of ointment of calendula extract in a neutral base showed a 41-percent decrease in total surface area of ulcers after three weeks. A control group whose ulcers were dressed with a saline solution showed a decrease in total ulcerous area of only 14 percent. Calendula can also be used to treat diaper dermatitis. It has been compared with aloe vera in treating diaper rash, and calendula achieved significantly better results. In addition to topical applications, calendula is packed with antioxidants and can be used internally for irritated or damaged digestive tissue.

BLACK PEPPER *Piper nigrum*

Using spices to increase digestive efficiency and nutrient absorption can also be helpful for the skin, bones, and joints. Our bones are our foundation and are more malleable than many people realize. Rather than static building blocks, bones are constantly changing, rebuilding, and regenerating. Healthy bones are built by mining minerals from the food we eat, and it is critical that the body can glean and use what it needs from our food. Black pepper is a star in increasing bioavailability of bone-building ingredients in your food. Black pepper contains calcium and helps the body increase its uptake of calcium. (Some other spices with relatively high levels of calcium include sesame seeds, savory, dill, and basil.)

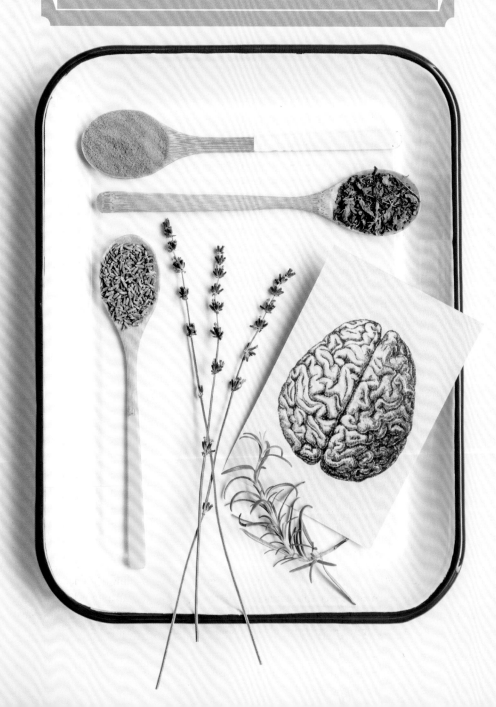

OFTENTIMES, INTERACTING with the world around us can send us into a tailspin as our nervous system reacts and responds to all the input. It's a rare person who doesn't feel they need a bit of help managing a busy life and routine stress, and staying above-water when things get difficult. These days, most of us need all the help we can get! Spices are invaluable tools to help bring ourselves back into balance.

Spices may not be the first thing you think of when it comes to achieving clarity and focus, but you might be surprised to learn how these flavorful additions to food can impact mental health and well-being. More and more, we are coming to recognize that certain mental health conditions are intimately connected with systemic inflammation — this is one way spices might fit into the picture. Additionally, there are a number of spices, such as rosemary, that have direct and acknowledged cognitive and neuroprotective effects.

Based on contemporary medical literature and a long history of healing traditions, intentionally using spices on a regular basis in your food can have significant effects on overall mental health, wellness, and disease prevention. This doesn't mean the use of spices can replace or supersede medications, but using nourishing, food-based spices that have antioxidant and anti-inflammatory properties may play a significant role in an overall path to wellness. The addition of spices to household meals can be invaluable for families with patterns of depression or anxiety.

One interesting mechanism we are continuing to learn about is the connection between the gut and the brain, often referred to as the gut-brain axis. Most people know that our brains can affect our guts. We know that when we are scared or upset it can create negative reactions in our stomach and gastrointestinal tract. We know that chronic stress can change bowel function and even result in irritable bowel syndrome (IBS). However, not everyone is aware of how the health of our gut and gastrointestinal tract can impact our mental health. Inflammatory bowel conditions, or even acute episodes of gut imbalance, can have a profound effect on mental health and well-being. Using spices and herbs to calm and soothe digestion is a useful way of addressing mental health and well-being when the gut seems to be involved (see Strengthen Digestion on page 95).

LAVENDER
Lavandula angustifolia

There have been numerous studies in support of lavender extract having a positive effect on calming the nervous system. One study examined use of *Lavandula angustifolia* essential oil by women with demanding full-time jobs and the subjects reported improvements in sleep and quality of life. Moreover, subjects who used an essential oil blend of lavender, clary sage, and sweet marjoram had a significantly greater improvement in both measurable outcomes, suggesting a synergistic effect. Research on essential oil doesn't directly point to dietary application, but given the compelling evidence in aromatherapy, adding a small amount of lavender to your spice blends or desserts may have some benefit.

ROSEMARY *Rosmarinus officinalis*

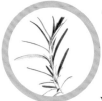

To support memory and overall cognitive function, adding rosemary to your diet is an excellent step. Its strong flavor, especially when fresh, is versatile, and an average cooking dose of even a half-teaspoon has notable medicinal benefits. Studies have shown that just a low dose of rosemary supports memory function. In one study, older adults (with a mean age of 75 years) received four different doses of *Rosmarinus officinalis*. The lowest dose (750 mg), a dose comparable to normal culinary consumption, significantly improved memory speed, while the highest dose (6,000 mg) impaired memory speed. Rosemary's essential oil also can be beneficial. It has been shown in one study to significantly enhance memory performance and alertness compared to lavender essential oil or placebo.

HOLY BASIL *Ocimum sanctum*

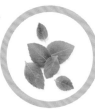

Holy basil is an adaptogen — a medicinal plant that supports the body's resilience against the impacts of stress. Adaptogens are some of the most widely used medicinal plants today, given our busy lifestyles and the levels of stress so many people experience. In one study examining the use of holy basil in treating patients with generalized anxiety disorder, patients were administered 500 mg of *Ocimum sanctum* extract twice daily. By the end of the trial the patients' anxiety, stress, and depressive symptoms had been significantly reduced. A 500 mg dose of holy basil extract, in this case, is about the same as you'd get in a typical food preparation, like eating a few leaves on a pizza or a tablespoon of pesto. In another study looking at the effects of holy basil on cognitive health, healthy adult participants were administered 300 mg capsules of holy basil leaf extract for 30 days. A number of cognitive improvements were noted, including fewer errors made while completing tasks and a reduction in the effects of cortisol stress levels. It's exciting to realize that one of the best adaptogens is so easy and delicious to add to our food on a daily basis.

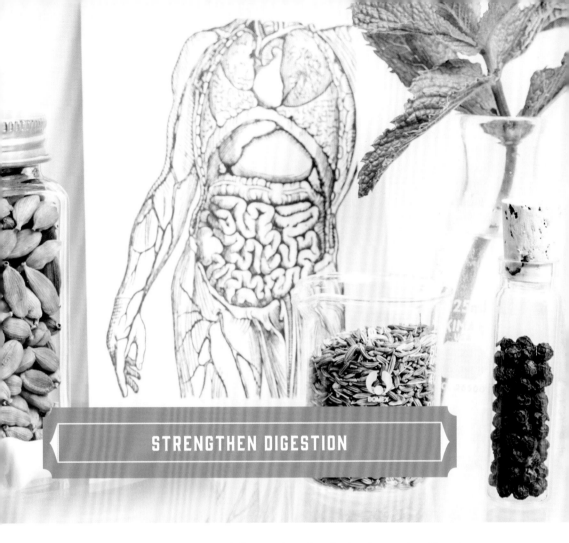

STRENGTHEN DIGESTION

WHILE MOST SPICES have beneficial digestive effects, a few really stand out. Peppermint, cardamom, black pepper, and fennel are four magnificent digestive spices. Their tastiness, diversity of use, and accessibility make them favorites worldwide.

Spices are integral to healthy digestion. As long as people have been cooking and preparing food, they have been using spices to add flavor, help preserve food, and aid digestion. Due to their aromatic principles, nearly all spices offer some sort of digestive benefit, whether increasing digestive secretions, optimizing digestive fire, reducing gas and bloating, or inducing satiety to prevent overeating. Our digestive system has a lot to contend with, dealing with all sorts of things we might throw at it. And, depending on its overall balance, it has a varying capacity to tackle these challenges.

The good news is, there are many herbs and spices that tonify your digestive tract and help with overall mucosal integrity and digestive capacity.

There is a possible link between cooking with spices and making healthy food choices in general. In one study, middle school kids were taught an educational curriculum about medicinal spices, then their food choices were tracked for a few months. Children who received training on spices continued to eat more vegetables and whole-grain carbohydrates after the study. It has also been shown that when eating generously spiced food (not spicy food, per se) people become fuller earlier and tended to eat less.

There are many ways to take spices when you're looking to optimize digestion. The most direct is to add them into food when cooking. Cardamom, fennel, and mint all work to settle the stomach and aid in digestion, and black pepper aids in absorption. You can also play around with these as digestifs, liquors, or teas.

There is evidence in support of black pepper being beneficial for tissue health. One study examined the use of black pepper in improving the health of oral mucosal tissue. After ingesting turmeric and black pepper for three months, patients with submucous fibrosis in the mouth experienced improvements in inflammation and a reduction in burning sensation. This is a good indication for the use of black pepper in stubborn conditions where there are blockages or fibrous tissue buildup. Another study of oral health showed that when patients with chronic periodontitis used an herbal mouthwash of black pepper, pomegranate rinds, and detoxified copper sulfate, it was determined to be as effective as a common prescription mouthwash in reducing the number of microorganisms and controlling chronic periodontitis noninvasively, with none of the side effects.

BLACK PEPPER *Piper nigrum*

One of the substances at work in black pepper is the alkaloid piperine, which works by stimulating the digestive enzymes of the pancreas. Piperine has shown a variety of effects in research, such as reducing transit time, increasing digestive capacity, and protecting against oxidative damage and stress. In higher doses, piperine can change the bioavailability of medications you take, which is something to consider. You can avoid this interaction in most cases by taking medications a few hours before or after you consume piperine.

MINT *Mentha* spp.

One clinical trial of the effect of peppermint oil for treating irritable bowel syndrome (IBS) showed significant improvement in symptoms. IBS patients received two peppermint oil capsules twice daily for four weeks and were evaluated for symptoms including abdominal bloating, pain or discomfort, diarrhea, constipation, feelings of incomplete evacuation, passage of gas or mucus, and urgency or pain at defecation. After four weeks, 75 percent of the group experienced a 50-percent or greater reduction of symptoms compared with only 38 percent of a placebo group. Clinical evidence suggests peppermint oil is modestly effective in reducing some common symptoms of IBS, especially flatulence and abdominal pain and distention, and may also be effective in treating non-ulcer dyspepsia. The one digestive symptom for which mint may not be helpful is regular gastric reflux. Mint works to loosen the esophageal sphincter to release gas and pressure from the gastrointestinal tract. In the case of acid reflux, however, this effect can be undesirable. If you are prone to gastric reflux, you can give mint a try to see how you respond to it.

FENNEL
Foeniculum vulgare

In one study, the essential oil of fennel seeds was determined to offer significant improvement in IBS symptoms and overall quality of life over the course of 30 days. As essential oil was used in this particular study, the results are not synonymous with the use of the seed itself. While essential oils are a significant part of the seed, there are some precautions to consider. In general, extracted essential oils contain a small percentage of the medicinal constituents available in a plant. An isolated essential oil has a specific targeted activity in the body. Additionally, given that essential oils contain a reasonably high dose of volatile oils, there is some amount of toxicity involved in all essential oils and they must be used in small amounts. By contrast, when using the fennel seed, either whole or ground, you get a complete profile of the medicinal constituents in a significantly safer form without any of the safety concerns that go along with essential oils.

CARDAMOM
Elettaria cardamomum

Cardamom is a warming carminative that dispels gas and bloating, improves digestion, and acts as an antispasmodic. Its flavor is sweet and palatable, although it needs to be used in small amounts, as it can be overpowering. Reducing stress and supporting the nervous system environment can, in turn, create calmer digestion. This doesn't mean that total nervous system serenity is necessary to have ideal digestion. If you have chronic or recurring digestive challenges of an idiopathic nature, you may also want to consider spices for your nervous system (see the Create Calm and Focus on page 92).

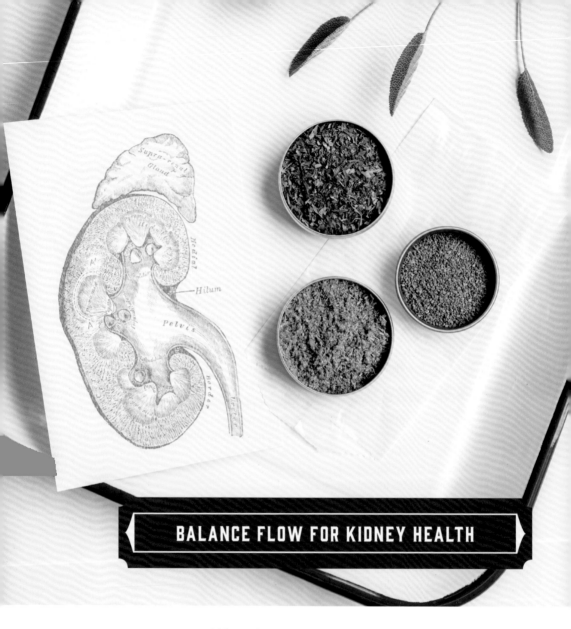

BALANCE FLOW FOR KIDNEY HEALTH

THE IMPORTANCE OF our kidneys is easy to forget until we have health challenges involving them. Our kidneys are connected to many different aspects of our health (or disease patterns), including blood pressure, kidney stones, gout, urinary tract infections, and other common conditions that can happen at different stages of life. Most of them require a variety of interventions to manage once present, especially later in life, so prevention is key.

Many chronic conditions involving the kidneys have deep roots, and preventive strategies offered through dietary spices are appropriate for those who have a family history of kidney issues. Individuals who have had kidney stones and want to prevent a reoccurrence, or those with hypertension or gout, may benefit from regular use of parsley, celery seed, and sage.

PARSLEY
Petroselinum crispum

Parsley is a wonderful kidney tonic and is incredibly helpful in nearly all conditions that impact the kidneys. It is a gentle diuretic and exhibits antimicrobial activity to help with mild urinary tract infections. It can also be helpful for individuals who tend to retain water and for those prone to developing kidney stones.

CELERY SEED
Apium graveolens

A small amount of celery seed proves quite effective in treating gout. This common ailment involving kidney health causes uric acid to pool in distal regions of the body — often in the feet, ankles, and toes — resulting in acute pain. While there are dietary and lifestyle considerations to address when someone is dealing with gout, celery seed can help optimize kidney function and uric acid excretion to alleviate the discomfort of gout.

SAGE *Salvia officinalis*

If you think of the body as an ocean, sage has the ability to act like a hot sun. Sage has been traditionally used to dry up excess or undesirable fluids produced by the body. For example, sage helps to dry up breast milk when ending lactation. It also decreases sweating, especially during menopausal hot flashes for which it has long been employed as a treatment. One study examined menopausal women, age 50 to 65, who were experiencing at least five hot flashes per day. They were given a sage extract of 250 mg daily (equivalent to 3.4 grams of fresh sage leaf), and, they kept a diary to record any changes in frequency and rate of intensity of hot flashes categorized as mild, moderate, severe, or very severe. Results showed an average 50-percent decrease in the number of flashes within the first four weeks and a 64-percent decrease by the end of eight weeks. In addition, the intensity of hot flashes decreased, including a 79-percent decrease in severe flashes and a 100-percent decrease in very severe flashes. The relative proportion of moderate, severe, and very severe hot flashes all decreased. A similar effect was demonstrated in a study that looked at hot flashes experienced by prostate cancer patients who had been treated with androgen deprivation. Note that if you already experience mucosal dryness, such as dry eyes or vaginal dryness, or you are a nursing mother, sage may not be the best spice for you.

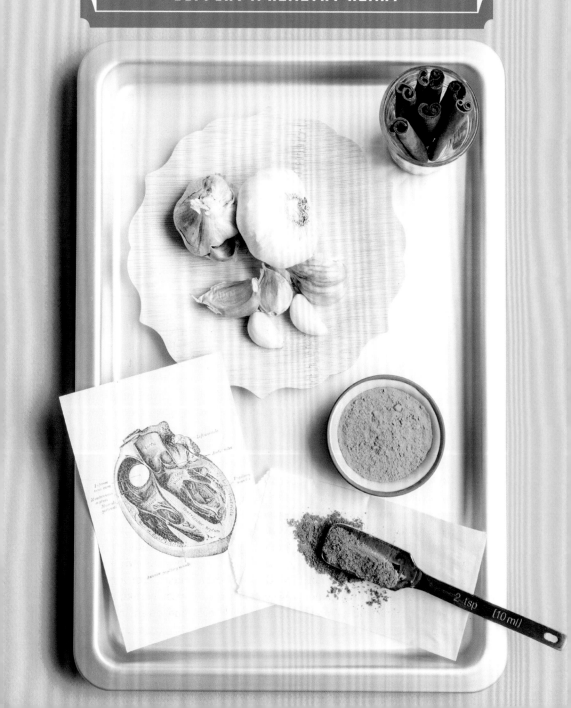

THE HUMAN POPULATION is experiencing epidemics of cardiovascular disease and related metabolic conditions. Adding a few spices to your diet might seem like a tiny sword to wield against heart disease, but you might be surprised at how effective it can be. Research shows that simple dietary additions of herbs and spices can have profound and lasting results on heart health. And most spices are compatible and safe to use alongside medications, so they do not limit medication options.

While many conditions involving the heart are genetic, others are passed from one generation to the next through lifestyle habits and life circumstances. Using spices can be part of a multi-generational approach to treating degenerative conditions. Adding spices to family meals can offer protection from developing certain diseases later in life and support optimal health in the process. Cinnamon, garlic, turmeric, and cumin are delicious additions to the pot when cooking for heart health.

CINNAMON *Cinnamomum* spp.

Cinnamon has been shown to help regulate blood glucose levels, which is specifically helpful in prediabetic individuals or those with concerns about diabetes. For people who are prediabetic or diabetic, cinnamon demonstrates beneficial activity when used alone or in conjunction with conventional pharmaceutical blood sugar management. Cinnamon is well tolerated, safe, generally liked, and easy to take. Even if you don't take cinnamon every day, studies suggest that regular dietary use — that is, incorporating it into your food — has a positive effect. Cinnamon appears to have a regulatory effect on blood glucose levels after eating even for people who are not diabetic or prediabetic.

In one study by the American Diabetes Association, varying doses of cinnamon were compared to placebo for several markers of metabolic syndrome, a cluster of biochemical and physiological abnormalities associated with the development of cardiovascular disease and type 2 diabetes. Patients were given doses of one, two, or three grams twice a day for 40 days. At the end of the trial, every group showed decreases in triglycerides, low-density lipoprotein (LDL) cholesterol, and total cholesterol. The largest amount of cinnamon did not always show the most change; the most improvement in triglyceride levels was seen among the 1-gram-per-day group, and the biggest changes in both total cholesterol and LDL were seen among the 2-gram-per-day group. So, more doesn't always mean better. It's best to just get in the habit of using cinnamon regularly.

GARLIC *Allium sativum*

Garlic deserves a place in every kitchen where there is concern for the heart. Garlic is a multifaceted mega-medicine for the cardiovascular system. In various meta-analyses of clinical trials, garlic has been shown to significantly lower total cholesterol levels over placebo. Over a two-year period, garlic, in aged extract form and given in conjunction with vitamins (B_{12}, B_6, and folic acid) and amino acid L-arginine, was studied for its ability to slow atherosclerosis progression. Atherosclerosis is an inflammatory condition where fatty deposits build up on the walls of the arteries. There was significant improvement in oxidative biomarkers among the group receiving garlic, with decreases in total cholesterol, LDL cholesterol, triglycerides, and C-reactive protein. In addition, there was an increase in high-density lipoprotein (HDL) cholesterol. These results show that garlic has benefits in retarding progression of atherosclerosis.

TURMERIC *Curcuma longa*

In a clinical trial studying the effects of curcumin, an active constituent of turmeric, on blood lipids, subjects had their blood serum levels measured and were then given 0.5 grams of curcumin per day for one week, after which blood lipid levels were reassessed. The results showed an average decrease in serum lipids of 33 percent, an average decrease in total cholesterol of 11 percent, an average decrease in triglycerides of 7 percent, and an average increase in HDL of 29 percent. This modest dose can be easily ingested by using a teaspoon of turmeric daily in food. To ensure bioavailability, turmeric is best when combined with black pepper and high-quality fats.

Curcumin has also been shown to halt the progression from prediabetes to type 2 diabetes mellitus (T2DM). Commonly, when people are diagnosed with prediabetes their goal is to prevent progression to diabetes through recommended dietary, pharmaceutical, and lifestyle strategies. One study examined the role of curcumin alone on prediabetic individuals. Participants were assessed for various markers of the disease and then given a daily dose of curcumin (250 mg of curcuminoids) or placebo and were reassessed every three months until the trial's conclusion. After nine months, results showed a significant improvement in markers among the curcumin group: the oral glucose tolerance test, fasting plasma glucose, hemoglobin A1c, c-peptide, and homeostatic model assessment of insulin resistance had all decreased in the curcumin group but increased or remained static in the placebo group. The homeostatic model assessment of beta cell function had increased in the curcumin group but decreased in the placebo group. At the end of nine months, 16 percent of the placebo group had progressed to a diagnosis of T2DM, but none of the curcumin group had!

CUMIN *Cuminum cyminum*

In one clinical trial, 78 overweight subjects aged 18 to 60 years old received either cumin capsules, a prescription weight loss drug, or a placebo three times a day for 8 weeks. At the end of the trial, the groups who consumed the cumin seed and those who took the pharmaceutical drug showed similar significant decreases in weight and body mass index (BMI) as compared with the placebo. Taking cumin also led to a significant reduction in blood serum insulin levels.

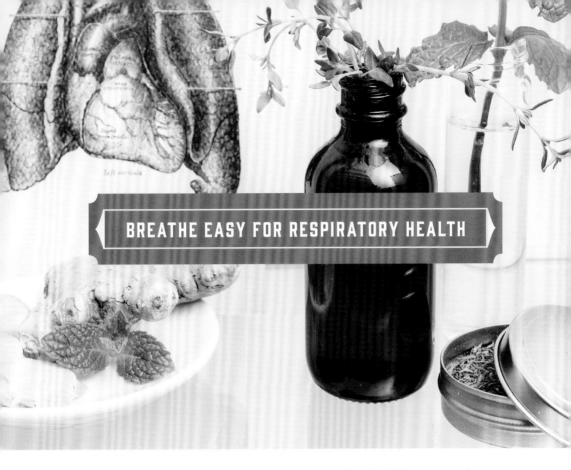

BREATHE EASY FOR RESPIRATORY HEALTH

IF YOU HAVE a respiratory infection, a touch of congestion, allergies, or asthma, spices may not be the first intervention you think of, but there is a long history of using certain spices for respiratory care. Mint, thyme, and ginger all help increase circulation, decrease inflammation, and support endogenous detoxification processes, which can be helpful in supporting respiratory wellness.

There are a few different ways to use spices to support the respiratory system. Dietary use in food and drink is effective for a broad preventive approach, as well as for treating acute conditions. Hot water extractions, or infused teas, can be

therapeutic. A cup of hot peppermint tea helps respiratory congestion caused by seasonal pollen.

MINT *Mentha* spp.

Of all the different mints, peppermint is preferred for respiratory health. Peppermint is packed with aromatic oils and can be wonderful for a variety of bronchial conditions. Using it as tea or as a steam are the most effective methods. Peppermint is a common constituent in chest balms and vapor rubs used to treat congestion. Making some peppermint tea in your kitchen will fill the air with anti-microbial and expectorant essential oils. A cup of peppermint tea can have a gentle clearing and expectorant action when you are congested from allergies or a cold or flu. It's also a good daily tonic to have on hand for people who experience asthma.

Topical approaches like steams can also be effective in reaching the lungs. Steams deliver the benefit of a spice directly to your lungs. They can be wonderful in situations of respiratory inflammation or congestion.

Some of the best spices to use for herbal steams are thyme, peppermint, and ginger (rosemary, sage, and fennel are also good choices). Any of these, used on their own or in a blend, can be appropriate and helpful. I have seen essential oils recommended for respiratory health, but I find they can be difficult to breathe in and can easily burn or irritate the eyes and skin. Using spices in a steam is safer, gentler, less expensive, and easier to have on hand when needed.

To create a respiratory steam, you'll need the spice or spice blend, a large bowl for hot water, and a towel. Put the bowl on a table where you can comfortably pull up a chair and sit in front of it. Boil about 2 cups of water and pour it into the bowl. Put about 1 tablespoon of the spice in to the bowl. Breathe in the steam as soon as it feels safe to do so. Be careful — steam can be very hot initially and can burn your skin. If you are working with a child, be sure to test the steam temperature with your own skin and let the child know when it is safe. When you are comfortable with the temperature, drape the towel over your head to trap the steam, and breathe it in for a few minutes.

GINGER
Zingiber officinale

There is some research on the antimicrobial effects of ginger in respiratory conditions. One in vitro study looked at the effects of ginger on antibiotic-resistant respiratory pathogens collected from throat swabs of patients with respiratory tract infections. The samples were taken of patients exhibiting symptoms of nasal discharge (runny nose), cough, or catarrh (excess mucus). Four different pathogens were isolated in the samples, and the strains were found to be resistant to five out of seven antibiotics, with only the two most expensive antibiotics being effective. In comparison, when ginger extracts were used to test each organism, the ginger extract exhibited antibacterial activity against all four pathogens. If you are dealing with respiratory infection specifically, see the discussion in Bolster Immune Protection and Defense (page 84) regarding antimicrobials.

Ginger works well in the case of stuck or stubborn mucus. This pungent rhizome acts as a "mover" — more so than a classic expectorant — and its warming nature makes it a good choice when the body is experiencing a cold or stagnant pattern. Using fresh ginger will offer balance, as it is both moist and warming, perfect as a tonic for the lungs. Dried ginger is both hot and dry, which can be a tricky combination when you are working to nurture or heal irritated lung tissue, as the lungs are naturally moist and you don't want to dry them out. Ginger tea, made by boiling slices of fresh ginger for about 10 minutes, is one of the best uses of ginger for respiratory support. Any food-based method that involves plenty of fresh grated ginger is also a great choice, such as Hot Ginger Lemonade (page 152) or Spicy Wonder Gingerbread (page 123).

Ginger has also shown positive results in cases of more serious respiratory ailments involving infectious disease. In a study examining its use in pulmonary tuberculosis, patients undergoing standard anti-tubercular treatment were randomly assigned to receive 3 grams of ginger or placebo daily for one month. A number of inflammatory markers (primary indications of the disease) were significantly reduced in the ginger group compared to the placebo group, confirming ginger's anti-inflammatory and antioxidant actions.

THYME
Thymus vulgaris

All of the Mediterranean aromatic herbs have extensive antimicrobial action, which is especially helpful for dealing with the respiratory system. Thyme, sage, rosemary, and oregano can all be used to support respiratory health — and they're even better used together. These herbs are effective when congestion of a possibly infectious origin is present, or for active respiratory sickness.

The expectorant activity of thyme was studied in a clinical trial of patients with bronchitis. Patients demonstrated a minimum of 10 daytime coughing episodes with an impaired ability to cough up mucus. They were then assigned an 11-day course of thyme and ivy leaf syrup taken three times per day for a total of 16.2 mL per day, with the syrup containing 15 percent thyme leaf extract and 1.5 percent ivy leaf extract. The average reduction in coughing episodes for the thyme group was 68 percent compared to a placebo group, and a 50-percent reduction in coughing episodes was reached two days sooner with the thyme group. Furthermore, the overall regression of symptoms was faster with the thyme group than the placebo group.

SPICES FOR SPECIFIC HEALTH CONCERNS

	BLACK PEPPER	CALENDULA	CARDAMON	CELERY SEED	CHILES	CINNAMON	CUMIN	FENNEL	GARLIC
ANXIETY & DEPRESSION									
CARDIOVASCULAR					X	X	X		X
CHOLESTEROL						X	X		X
DIABETES					X	X	X		X
DIGESTIVE SUPPORT FOR KIDS			X				X	X	
GASTRIC TONIC	X		X		X	X	X	X	
GOUT		X		X					
HOT FLASHES									
HYPERTENSION									X
IMMUNE SUPPORT					X				X
INFECTION		X							X
INFLAMMATION		X			X	X			X
JOINT DISEASE	X				X	X			
KIDNEY TONIC		X		X					
MEMORY	X						X		
NEURO PROTECTION							X		
ORAL HEALTH	X	X							
RESPIRATORY INFECTION		X			X				X
RESPIRATORY TONIC		X							
SATIETY					X				
SKIN HEALTH AND HEALING		X							
STRESS MANAGEMENT									

GINGER	HOLY BASIL	LAVENDER	MINT	MUSTARD	PARSLEY	ROSEMARY	SAGE	THYME	TURMERIC
	X	X	X			X			X
X	X			X		X			X
X	X			X					X
X	X								X
X			X						
X			X	X					X
	X			X	X		X		
	X	X	X			X	X		
		X			X				X
X	X			X					X
X	X						X	X	X
X	X	X	X	X		X			X
X									X
					X		X		
	X	X	X	X		X			
X	X	X				X			X
							X	X	X
X			X	X		X	X	X	X
X	X		X	X		X		X	
		X							X
	X	X	X			X			

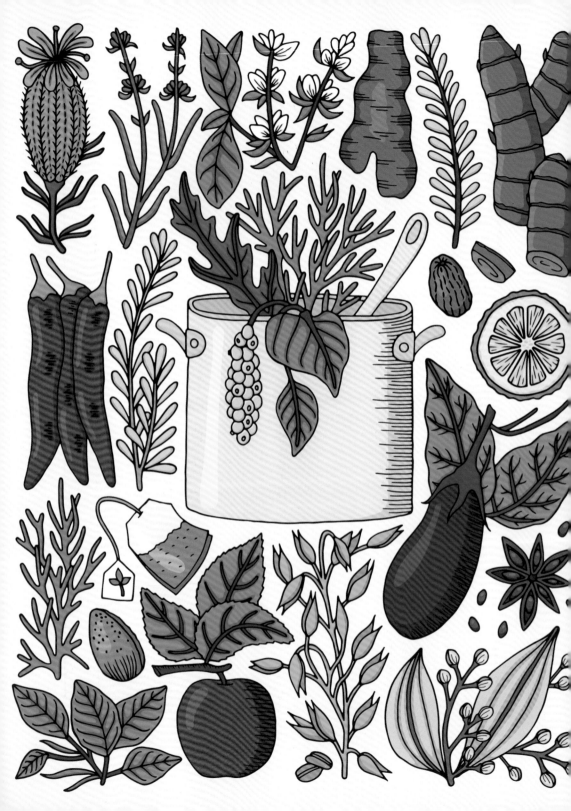

CHAPTER 5

Recipes

Creating dried spice blends is a simple way to fill your life with spices without too much hassle. Starting with the spice blends in this chapter, you can experiment and explore, swapping out or adding spices for your taste or desired therapeutic action. You'll also find some suggestions for using spice blends in foods as well as a few easy recipes featuring fresh herbs and spices.

A LITTLE SPICE EVERY DAY

There aren't a lot of hard-and-fast rules when using medicinal spices for health. As long as you are taking enough of a daily dose to have an effect, the way you consume them, which spices you consume, and how long you use them can vary. The recipes here are ideas and jumping-off points for you to begin using spices in your daily routine. Feel free to play around, substitute, add, subtract, or modify them. My main recommendation is to get a little bit of spice every day over a long period of time. Once you have a spice blend made, it becomes very easy to throw it in your cookpot or add it to a fresh recipe.

BLENDING SPICES

For centuries, certain spices have been combined to create blends that are both delicious and healing. Many of them are familiar — like cinnamon and clove in a fall pie, or garlic, basil, and oregano in Italian dishes — but the art of blending spices requires some know-how.

BLENDING FOR FLAVOR

Knowing which flavors truly suit each other requires either a highly skilled palate or a familiarity with the traditions of cuisine within a culture. Without a good foundation of knowledge about the flavors and behaviors of each spice, it can be difficult to imagine how they will pair. But there are some easy guidelines. For example, spices and herbs that are native to a certain region or have been used together traditionally in cooking usually make excellent companions.

If you want to get started blending herbs and spices, it's smart to look to the region of the world where the dish you are making — or your favorite cuisine — originates. Often, the spices that are native to a region are also frequently used in traditional dishes of that region. There are also a number of spices — notably garlic, ginger, chiles, and peppercorns — that have traveled the globe and now show up prominently in cuisines around the world. Choosing a few spices from one region or one cuisine is a good place to start when experimenting with spices that might pair well in a blend.

BLENDING FOR HEALTH GOALS

If your goal is to add a specific herb or spice into your diet for health benefits, you'll want to consider the nature of the spice. Is it sweet, spicy, pungent, or bitter? Does it cause a warming effect in your body when you eat it (like peppers, garlic, or ginger), or maybe a cooling and soothing effect (like mint and calendula)? Look for similar or complementary flavors. Tuning into these kinds of attributes of the spice can be a good way to get to know which spices might work well together in a blend. For more about spices that address specific health goals, see page 106.

You can also look to native spices (page 6) and spices used in regional cuisines (page 112). For example, if you are trying to consume regular amounts of turmeric, note that it is commonly used on the Indian subcontinent and would likely pair well with other spices native to or traditionally used in the region, like cumin, ginger, chile, and garlic. Don't be afraid to get creative and try new things. Blend small amounts to start and take notes on how things are working. Remember, you may get the best flavors when you cook a blend into your food. Above all, enjoy playing with blends and the way they come together, and be open to discovering new combinations you love!

DRIED SPICE BLENDS

Blends of dried spices can be an excellent way to increase your overall consumption of spices, or to ensure you get a therapeutic dose of a particular spice. When we are in a rush or don't have access to fresh spices, grabbing a jar or a bag of a favorite blend is easy and effective. Spice blends can be added to food while cooking, and many of these blends can even be added to already prepared foods. I like to keep shaker jars of my favorite blends on my kitchen table to sprinkle on top of whatever I'm eating.

When creating dried spice blends, it's ideal to use all the spices in the blend in the same form. So, all in powder form or all in cut-and-sifted form. However, some dried spices are available only as a powder, such as ginger. If you're making a cut-and-sifted mixture and want to use ginger, that's okay. Just know that the powdered spice will sink to the bottom of the jar or bag, so it's important to give the container a good shake or stir before using.

USING SPICE BLENDS IN FOODS

Spices can elevate a dish from mundane to something fabulous and memorable. While fresh spices are always a delight, they can be difficult or expensive to get at certain times of the year. Dried spices offer a wide selection and are easy to keep on hand for daily meals. Cultures around the world have used spice blends to create unique and iconic dishes, and it's not hard for you to do the same. When added to food, spice blends pack a medicinal punch along with delicious flavor.

While it is preferable to discuss dosing with spices for health benefits in terms of grams per day, unless you have a digital scale that can measure partial grams, most people find it easier to use teaspoon and tablespoon measurements for cooking. However, teaspoon and tablespoon doses can vary widely depending on the format of the herb you are measuring, especially if you are using a cut variety versus a powdered preparation. For the sake of ease and simplicity, the Medicinal Use and Dosage chart (page 80) recommends a therapeutic daily dose for each spice in grams and also provides you with the approximate teaspoon or tablespoon equivalent.

GLOBAL FLAVOR PROFILES FOR BLENDING SPICES

NORTH AMERICAN COMMON BLENDS

Barbeque, Cajun

TRY THESE

ALLSPICE
ANNATTO
BAY
CHILES
CITRUS
COCOA
CUMIN
DILL
EPAZOTE
GARLIC
JUNIPER
ONION
OREGANO
PEPPERCORN
SASSAFRAS
VANILLA

CARIBBEAN COMMON BLENDS

Jerk, West Indies curries

TRY THESE

ALLSPICE
CARDAMOM
CHILES
CINNAMON
CLOVE
GARLIC
GINGER
MACE
NUTMEG
PEPPERCORNS
THYME

LATIN AMERICAN COMMON BLENDS

Mole
(green, red,
black, brown),
Chili powder

TRY THESE:

ALLSPICE
ANNATTO
BAY
CHILES
CILANTRO
CITRUS
CLOVES
COCOA
CORIANDER
CUMIN
EPAZOTE
GARLIC
OREGANO
PEPPERCORNS
VANILLA

AFRICAN COMMON BLENDS

Dukkah, Ras el hanout,
Berbere

TRY THESE

AJWAIN
ANISE
ASAFETIDA
BARBERRY
CARDAMOM
CUBEB PEPPER
CUMIN
GRAINS OF PARADISE
LONG PEPPER
NIGELLA
SESAME
TAMARIND

NORTHERN AND CENTRAL EUROPEAN COMMON BLENDS

Bouquet garni,
Fines herbes

TRY THESE

BAY
CARAWAY
CARDAMOM
CELERY SEED
CHERVIL
CHIVES
CINNAMON
CLOVE
CORIANDER
DILL
FENNEL
FENUGREEK
GARLIC
GINGER
HORSERADISH
JUNIPER
MINT
NUTMEG
ORANGE PEEL
PAPRIKA
PEPPERCORNS
POPPY SEED
SAFFRON
STAR ANISE
TARRAGON

MEDITERRANEAN COMMON BLENDS

Bharat, Ras el hanout

TRY THESE

ANISE
BASIL
BAY
CHIVES
FENNEL
FENUGREEK
GARLIC
LAVENDER
MARJORAM
MINT
MUSTARD
OREGANO
PARSLEY
PEPPERCORNS
ROSEMARY
SAFFRON
SAGE
TARRAGON
THYME

SOUTH PACIFIC COMMON BLENDS

Chili powder, Chinese five spice, Garam masala

TRY THESE

CHILES
CORIANDER
GALANGAL
GARLIC
GINGER
TAMARIND
TURMERIC

MIDDLE EASTERN COMMON BLENDS

Za'atar

TRY THESE

ALLSPICE
BLACK CUMIN
CARAWAY
CARDAMOM
CINNAMON
CLOVES
CUMIN
GARLIC
GINGER
MINT
NIGELLA
NUTMEG
OREGANO
PARSLEY
PEPPERCORNS
SAFFRON
SESAME
SUMAC
THYME
TURMERIC

INDIAN SUBCONTINENT COMMON BLENDS

Tumeric-based curries, Vindaloo

TRY THESE

AJWAIN
ALLSPICE
ASAFETIDA
BAY
CARDAMOM
CHILES
CINNAMON
CITRUS PEEL
CLOVE
CORIANDER

INDIAN SUBCONTINENT, *CONTINUED*

CUMIN
FENNEL
FENUGREEK
GARLIC
GINGER
MINT
MUSTARD
PEPPERCORNS
SESAME
TURMERIC

ASIAN COMMON BLENDS

Green, yellow, red, and massaman curry paste blends

TRY THESE

BASIL
CHILES
CILANTRO
CINNAMON
CITRUS PEEL
CLOVES
CORIANDER
GALANGAL
GARLIC
GINGER
LEMONGRASS
MUSTARD
PEPPERCORNS
SESAME
STAR ANISE
TAMARIND
WASABI

MEASURING IN PARTS

The dried spice blend recipes in this book use a technique, common in herbal medicine, of measuring in parts. It's a scalable and proportional way to easily make as little or as much of the blend as you want. Each "part" is equivalent to one measuring unit of your choice. For example, if a blend calls for 2 parts dried basil, 2 parts dried parsley, and 1 part garlic powder — and you decide you want to make a large amount of the blend — you could choose a half-cup as your "part" measure. So, if the recipe calls for 2 parts dried basil, you would use 2 half-cups of basil (1 cup total), the same of dried parsley, and then 1 half-cup of garlic powder. If you wanted to make a smaller amount of the blend, you might choose a teaspoon as your "part" measure. In this case, you would use 2 teaspoons of basil, 2 teaspoons of parsley, and 1 teaspoon of garlic. Basically, the recipes are a guide for creating a blend with the right proportions of each spice.

SCALABLE PARTS

SPICE	WRITTEN AS PARTS	TO MAKE A SMALL AMOUNT	TO MAKE A LARGE AMOUNT
BASIL LEAF	2 parts	2 teaspoons	2 x half-cups (1 cup total)
PARSLEY LEAF	2 parts	2 teaspoons	2 x half-cups (1 cup total)
GARLIC POWDER	1 part	1 teaspoon	½ cup
TOTAL BLEND	N/A	5 teaspoons	2½ cups

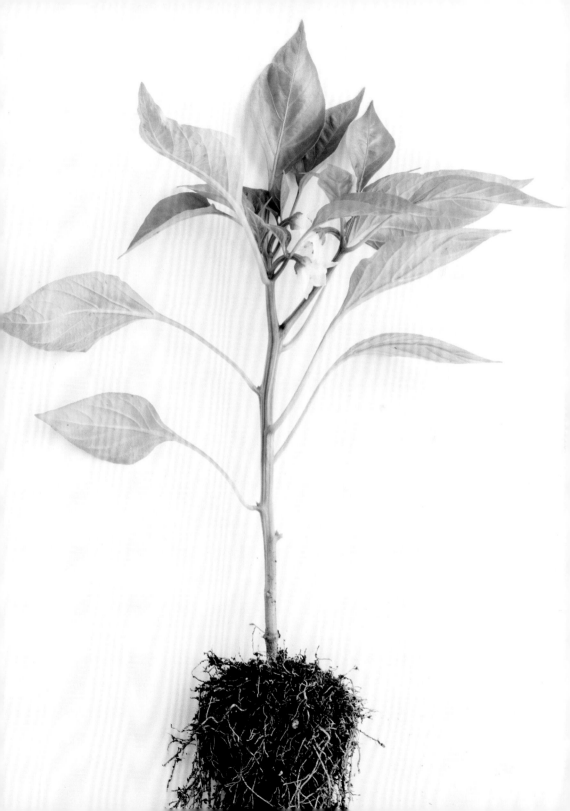

Everyday on Everything Blend

Overall tonic, acts as an anti-inflammatory, supports heart health, supports kidney health, supports respiratory health

Delicious on nearly anything savory, this blend can be used during cooking or can be sprinkled right on top of a finished dish. It's a perfect blend to keep in a jar on your table. It's versatile and forgiving, so feel free to leave out any ingredients you aren't crazy about. One of my favorite ways to use this is to mix it into eggs when making an omelet.

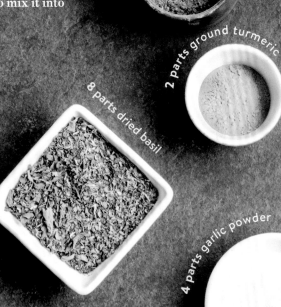

2 parts dried rosemary

2 parts dried sage

2 parts ground turmeric

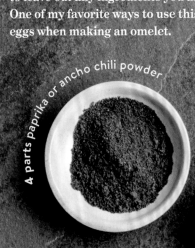

4 parts paprika or ancho chili powder

8 parts dried basil

4 parts garlic powder

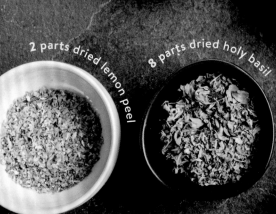

2 parts dried lemon peel

8 parts dried holy basil

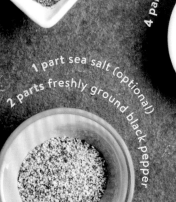

1 part sea salt (optional)

2 parts freshly ground black pepper

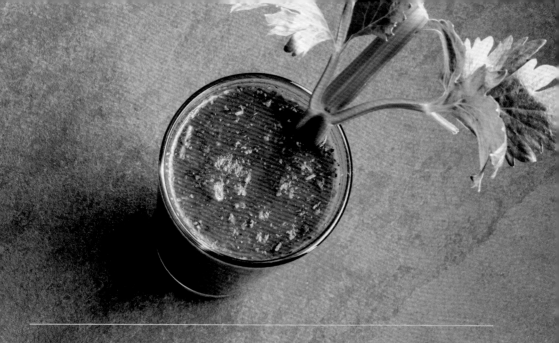

SPICY VIRGIN BLOODY MARY

Yield: 1 serving
Dose per serving: black pepper 1.3 grams | dried basil 1.2 grams | garlic 3.0 grams |
holy basil 1.2 grams | paprika or ancho chile 2.6 grams | rosemary 0.7 grams |
sage 0.4 grams | turmeric 1.2 grams

You might be surprised at how many medicinal spices you can pack into a glass of tomato
juice! This nonalcoholic version of a classic Bloody Mary can be spiced up or down as
you like.

2 tablespoons
Everyday on
Everything Blend

16 ounces tomato
juice (or other
vegetable juice
blend)

Hot sauce
(optional)

Celery, cherry
tomato, or
cucumber for
garnish (optional)

1. Stir 2 tablespoons of the Everyday on Everything
   Blend into the tomato juice, adding more to taste.

2. Add the hot sauce to taste, if using, and pour the
   mixture into glasses.

3. Garnish each glass with celery or other garnish,
   if desired, and serve.

HERBY GRAVY

Yield: 6 servings
Dose per serving: black pepper 0.1 grams | chile 0.23 grams | garlic 0.25 grams
holy basil 0.1 grams | rosemary 0.07 grams | sage 0.03 grams | turmeric 0.1 grams

This rich and savory gravy uses olive oil and spices to create a flavor-packed sauce
to pour over meats, tofu, or a batch of mashed root vegetables.

¼ cup butter or
olive oil

1 medium onion,
finely diced

¼ cup unbleached
all-purpose flour
or oat flour

3 cups vegetable
or chicken broth

2 tablespoons
soy sauce or tamari

1 tablespoon
Worcestershire
sauce

1 tablespoon
Everyday on
Everything Blend

¼ teaspoon freshly
ground black
pepper

1. Melt half of the butter in a saucepan over medium
   heat. Add the onion and cook for about 12 minutes,
   until the onion begins to brown. Add the remaining
   butter and allow to melt. Gradually add the flour,
   stirring to be sure it doesn't stick to the bottom of the
   pan, until the onions are coated, and continue to cook
   for about 30 seconds.

2. Add the broth, the soy sauce, the Worcestershire sauce,
   and the Everyday on Everything Blend, and whisk
   until the mixture comes to a simmer. Continue to whisk
   for about 10 minutes or until desired consistency is
   reached. Season with salt and pepper to taste and
   serve immediately.

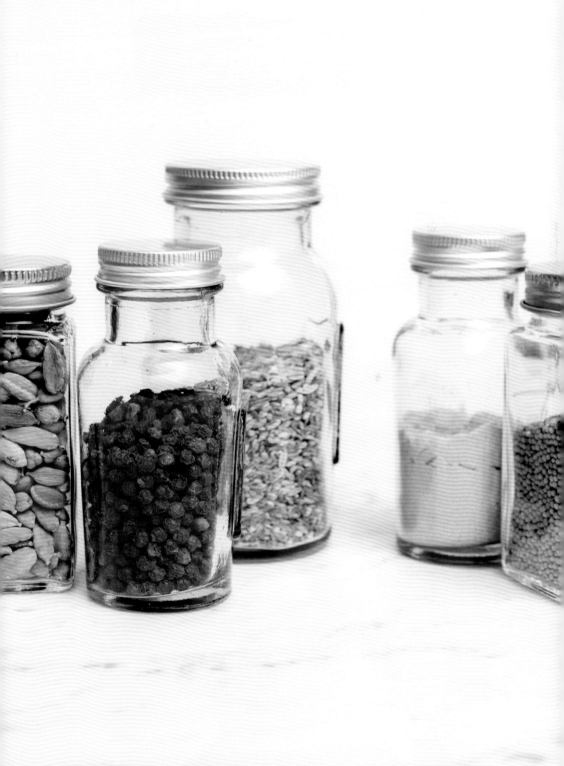

Reminds-Me-of-Pie Blend

Supports heart health, stabilizes blood sugar, warms digestion

The spices commonly found in delicious fall foods like apple crisp and pumpkin pie offer significant cardiovascular benefits. This blend maximizes the medicine of cinnamon and ginger and there are endless ways to use it. Try adding it to your morning oatmeal or yogurt, using it in pumpkin pie, sprinkling it on sweet potatoes, or spooning some into a latte or warm almond milk.

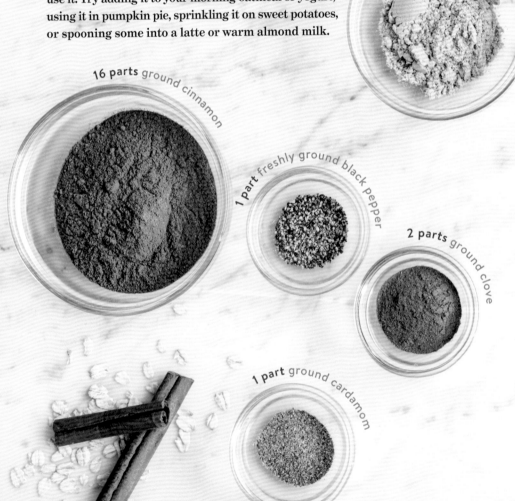

4 parts ground ginger

16 parts ground cinnamon

1 part freshly ground black pepper

2 parts ground clove

1 part ground cardamom

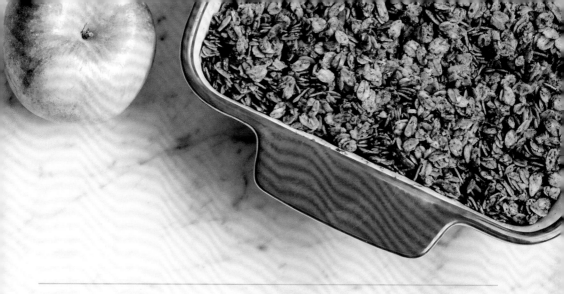

CINNAMON APPLE OAT BAKE

Yield: 4 servings
Dose per serving: black pepper 0.4 grams | cardamom 3.3 grams | cinnamon 3.9 grams | clove 0.5 grams | ginger 1.1 grams

This not-too-sweet apple and oat bake is perfect as a healthy dessert or topped with yogurt for a delicious breakfast. You can add more oats for a heartier dish.

3 tablespoons Reminds-Me-of-Pie Blend

3 tablespoons maple syrup

8 apples sliced into wedges (peeled if you want) with cores removed

2 cups rolled oats

½ teaspoon salt

½ cup melted coconut oil or butter

1. Adjust an oven rack to the center position and preheat the oven to 350°F (175°C). Grease an 8-inch square baking dish.

2. In a large bowl, toss the apples with 1 tablespoon of the Reminds-Me-of-Pie Blend and 1 tablespoon of the maple syrup. Pour the mixture into the prepared baking dish and spread evenly.

3. Combine the oats, salt, and the remaining 2 tablespoons of the Reminds-Me-of-Pie Blend in the now-empty bowl and mix well. Add the oil and the remaining 2 tablespoons of the maple syrup and stir until blended.

4. Spread the oat mixture onto the apple mixture and bake for 25 to 30 minutes, until the topping is golden and the apples are soft. Serve warm or cold.

CINNAMON SPICE JELLIES

Yield: 4 servings
**Dose per serving: black pepper 0.25 grams | cardamom 0.2 grams |
cinnamon 2.6 grams | ginger 0.75 grams**

These jiggly jelly candies are healthy and made with natural ingredients. Play around with
adding different spices, juices, or fruits — so fun!

1 cup apple cider or
 unfiltered apple
 juice

1½ tablespoons
 unflavored gelatin
 or agar-agar

2 tablespoons
 Reminds-Me-of-Pie
 Blend

1. Warm the cider in a small saucepan over medium heat
 until it boils. Off heat, whisk in the gelatin until it is
 completely dissolved. Stir in the Reminds-Me-of-Pie
 Blend.

2. Pour mixture into a 4-inch round or square baking
 dish or silicone mold. Refrigerate for at least 2 hours,
 until fully set. Slice into cubes or use cookie cutters to
 create shapes. Serve chilled or store in the refrigerator.

SPICY WONDER GINGERBREAD

Yield: 6 servings
Dose per serving: black pepper 0.12 grams | cardamom 0.1 grams | cinnamon 1.15 grams | ginger 2 grams | mustard 1 gram

More spicy than sweet, this gingerbread tickles the tongue! It's amazing as a dessert with fresh whipped cream on top.

6 tablespoons butter

⅓ cup grated fresh gingerroot

½ cup molasses

¼ cup honey

1 cup plain whole milk yogurt

1 egg

1 cup unbleached all-purpose flour

1 cup whole wheat flour or oat flour

4 teaspoons Reminds-Me-of-Pie Blend

1½ teaspoons baking soda

1 teaspoon ground mustard

¼ teaspoon salt

1. Adjust an oven rack to the center position and preheat the oven to 350°F (175°C). Grease an 8-inch square baking pan.

2. In a small skillet, melt the butter over medium low heat. Sauté the ginger until fragrant but not browned. Set aside to cool.

3. In a small bowl, beat the molasses and the honey with a hand mixer on high speed until well combined, 2 to 3 minutes. Add the yogurt and the egg, and beat until well blended, 2 minutes more. Add the cooled butter-and-ginger mixture.

4. In a large bowl, whisk together the all-purpose flour, whole wheat flour, Reminds-Me-of-Pie Blend, baking soda, mustard, and salt. Make a well in the center of the flour mixture and pour in the wet mixture. Mix, but be careful not to overmix as the gingerbread will turn out flat.

5. Spread the batter into the prepared pan. Bake for 30 to 35 minutes, until the top springs back when gently poked. Serve warm or cold.

Green Goodness Blend

Acts as an anti-inflammatory, supports heart health, supports kidney health, calms and nourishes

This blend is especially good when added to a creamy base to make a dip or dressing — you can use Greek yogurt, cream cheese, mayonnaise, buttermilk, sour cream, or even a vegan nut cheese. Use this by the handful rather than the teaspoon!

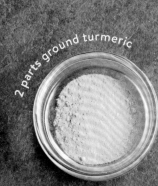

2 parts ground turmeric

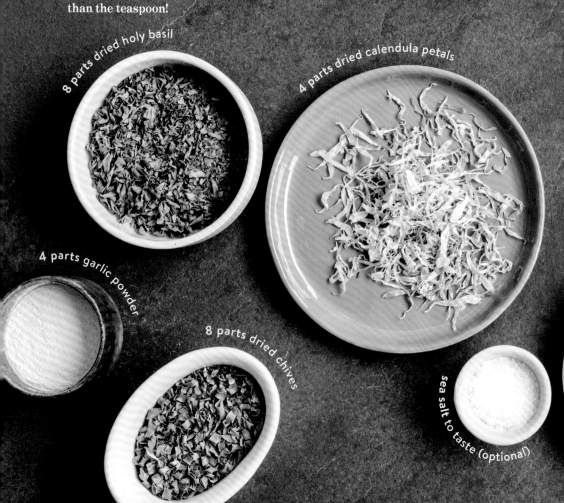

8 parts dried holy basil

4 parts dried calendula petals

4 parts garlic powder

8 parts dried chives

sea salt to taste (optional)

GREEN GOODNESS DRESSING

Yield: 1¼ cups
Daily Dose per batch: black pepper 0.6 grams |
calendula 0.3 grams | garlic 1.8 grams | holy basil 1 gram | parsley 0.8 grams |
turmeric 1 gram

This salad dressing is also a great dip for veggies or bread. If you're using yogurt,
a thicker variety like Greek yogurt is best. The optional grated cucumber transforms
it into a special spiced tzatziki sauce.

1   cup plain whole milk
    yogurt or labneh

1   cucumber, seeded and
    grated (optional)

2   tablespoons Green
    Goodness Blend

1   clove garlic, crushed
    (optional)

    Salt

Stir together the yogurt, the cucumber, if using, the
Green Goodness Blend, and the garlic, if using.
Refrigerate the mixture for 1 hour (or up to three
days) to allow flavors to meld. Season with salt to
taste and serve.

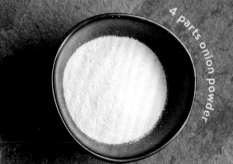

4 parts onion powder

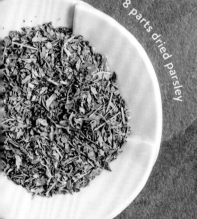

8 parts dried parsley

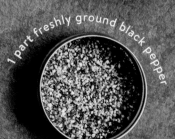

1 part freshly ground black pepper

Seed Blend

Warms digestion, acts as an anti-inflammatory, increases satiety, supports kidney health

Tiny seeds can pack quite a punch! They are wonderfully aromatic and warming and can create bold flavors. This blend can be left as whole seeds, crushed with a mortar and pestle, or blended into a powder for a smoother texture.

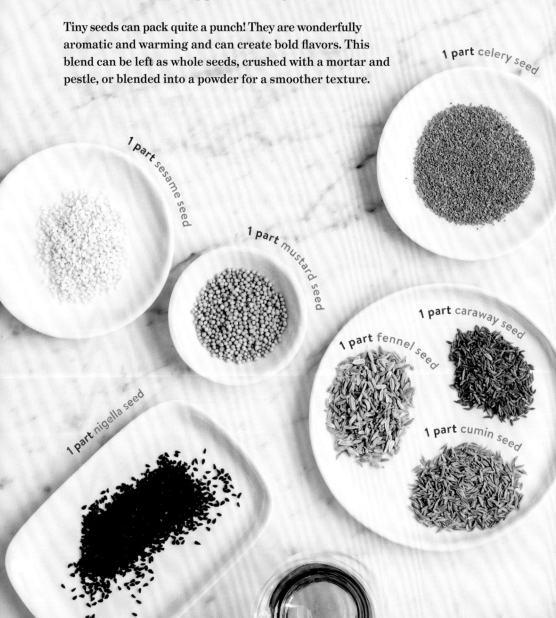

1 part celery seed

1 part sesame seed

1 part mustard seed

1 part caraway seed

1 part fennel seed

1 part cumin seed

1 part nigella seed

ROASTED EGGPLANT WITH GARLIC YOGURT

Yield: 4 servings

Dose per serving: celery 0.9 grams | cumin 0.9 grams | fennel 1 gram | mustard 0.8 grams

This roasted eggplant can be eaten as a side dish with meat or over rice and also makes a great dip.

1 large eggplant

4 tablespoons olive oil

1 large white onion

4 teaspoons Seed Blend

1 cup plain whole milk Greek yogurt, plus more for serving

2 cloves garlic, finely chopped or pressed

1 teaspoon apple cider vinegar

1. Adjust an oven rack to the middle position and preheat the oven to 400°F (200°C). Place the whole eggplant in a baking pan and rub it with 2 tablespoons of the oil. Roast for 45 minutes to 1 hour at 400°F (200°C), until it is soft and the skin begins to blister and char a bit.

2. Meanwhile, peel the onion and cut it into four thick slices, keeping the rings whole. Lay the rings on a greased baking sheet, drizzle with 1 tablespoon of the remaining oil, then top each slice with 1 teaspoon of the Seed Blend. Roast on the center rack for 30 to 45 minutes, until they are soft and slightly browned.

3. While the vegetables are roasting, combine the yogurt and the garlic and refrigerate to meld the flavors.

4. Allow the eggplant to cool slightly. Once it is cool enough to handle, slice the eggplant in half lengthwise and scrape the flesh, along with any accumulated juices, into a food processor or blender; discard the skin. Add the onions, along with any accumulated juices, the remaining 1 tablespoon oil, and the vinegar to the food processor and process until smooth, about 5 seconds. Transfer to a serving bowl, season with salt to taste, drizzle with additional yogurt, and serve warm.

Mint and Chile Blend

Warms digestion, prevents and treats gas and bloating, supports heart health

Mint and chiles make a blend of cool and hot. You can use whatever chiles you like. If you prefer something mild, use paprika or ancho chile. If you like heat, try cayenne or chipotle. I like to add this blend to yogurt and serve it with a curry or spicy grilled dish. It's also wonderful over couscous and vegetables. Dried mint doesn't have a very long shelf life, so don't store this blend for more than 3 months.

1 part dried mint

1 part chile flakes or powder

sea salt to taste (optional)

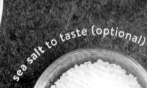

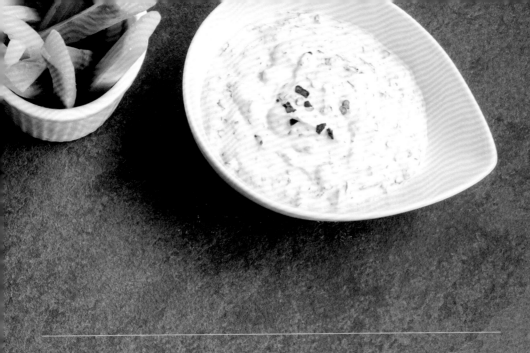

MINTY YOGURT SPREAD

Yield: 1¼ cups
Daily Dose per batch: chile 11.4 grams | mint 6.6 grams

This is lovely as a dip for fresh or roasted vegetables. You can also use it to top soups, stews, or spicy curries. Greek yogurt works well here.

1 cup plain whole milk yogurt, goat milk yogurt, or labneh

2 tablespoons Mint and Chile Blend

3 tablespoons fresh mint, finely chopped

Salt

In a small bowl, stir together the yogurt, the Mint and Chile Blend, and the mint. Let the mixture sit at room temperature or refrigerated for 30 minutes to allow the flavors to meld. Season with salt to taste and serve.

Warming Digestive Blend

Warms digestion, prevents and treats gas and bloating, relieves post-meal fatigue, relieves constipation, supports heart health

This sweet and warm blend is wonderful to try when you feel bloated or experience gas or constipation. It offers a lot of support to a recovering digestive system after illness or a dose of antibiotics. Plus, it's absolutely delicious!

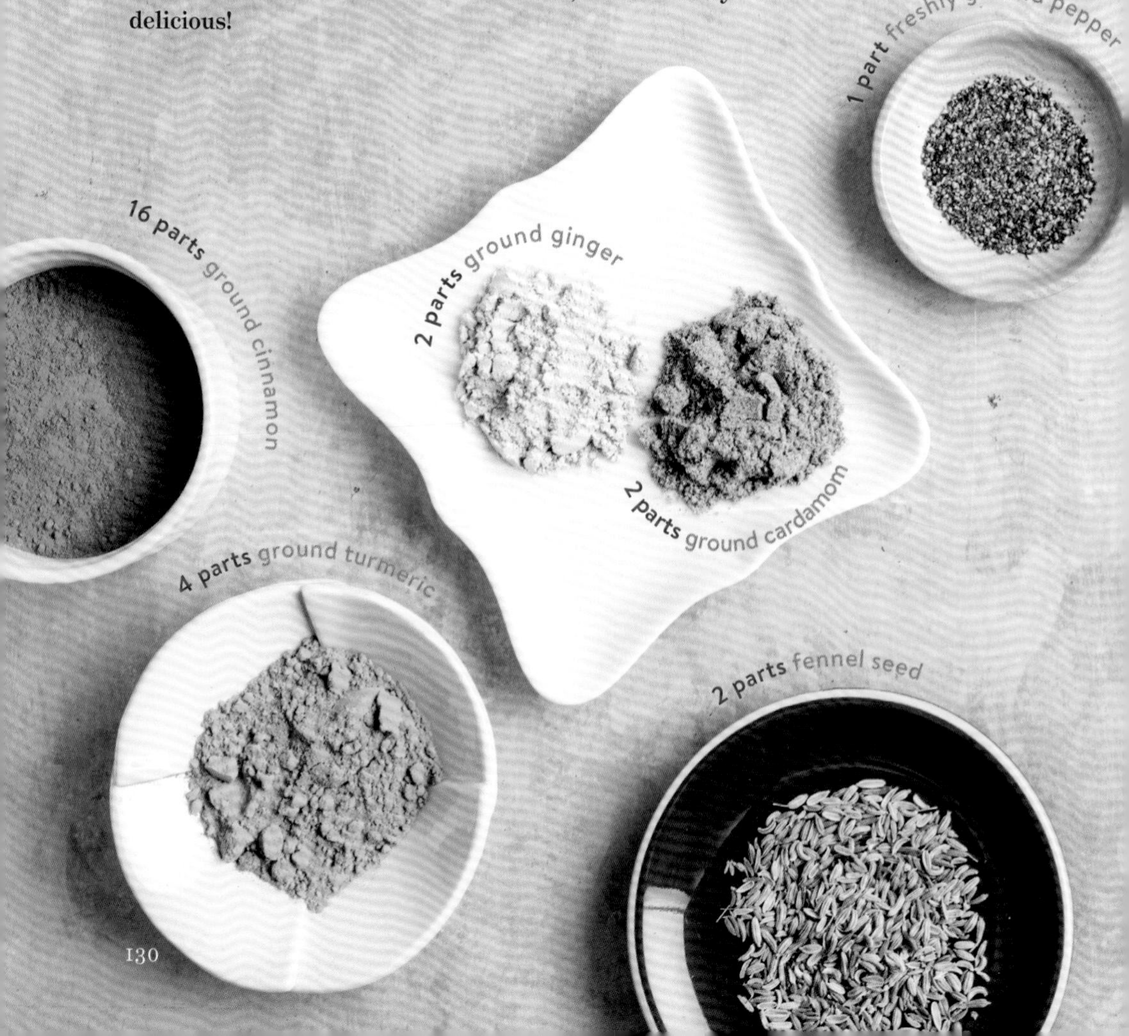

1 part freshly ground pepper

16 parts ground cinnamon

2 parts ground ginger

2 parts ground cardamom

4 parts ground turmeric

2 parts fennel seed

COMFY COMPOTE

Yield: 4 servings
Dose per serving: black pepper 0.1 grams | cardamom 0.2 grams | cinnamon 1.1 grams |
fennel 0.2 grams | ginger 0.2 grams | turmeric 0.4 grams

A balm for an irritated or unbalanced digestive system, the carminative spices in this
compote soothe inflammation and help with spasms and cramping. The fruits are good
for your gut bacteria. You can serve the compote warm or cold, alone or stirred into
yogurt or oatmeal. I like to make a big batch and freeze portions in small containers
as an easy grab when I need a little digestive support.

3 cups pitted and
 chopped fresh fruit
 (apples, cherries,
 apricots, peaches,
 pears, or plums)

1 cup dried fruit

1 tablespoon
 Warming Digestive
 Blend

2 tablespoons honey
 or sugar (optional)

In a small saucepan, stir together the fresh and dried
fruit and add enough water to cover the bottom of the
pan. Stir in the Warming Digestive Blend and cook,
covered, over medium-high heat, until the fruit is softened
but not completely mushy. Add sweetener if desired.
Remove from the heat and let cool slightly. Serve warm
or cold.

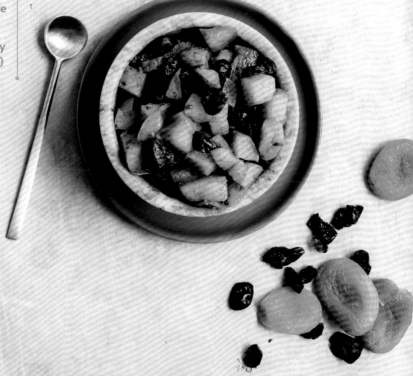

Fennel Dukkah Blend

Warms digestion, prevents and treats gas and bloating, relieves post-meal fatigue, relieves constipation, supports heart health

This savory blend is based on a traditional spice mixture commonly used in Egypt. It's wonderful mixed with a little olive oil or yogurt and used on salads or as a dip for pita bread. Careful — it can be a bit addicting! Giving it a few pulses in a food processor or spice grinder (or using a mortar and pestle) will crack the seeds and open up their flavors, but be careful not to overprocess it, as you don't want to make it into nut butter.

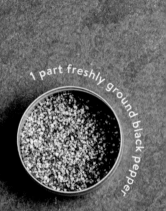

1 part freshly ground black pepper

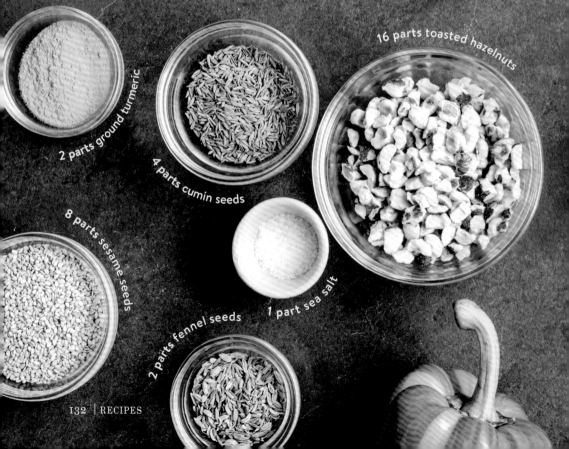

2 parts ground turmeric

4 parts cumin seeds

16 parts toasted hazelnuts

8 parts sesame seeds

1 part sea salt

2 parts fennel seeds

DUKKAH ROASTED VEGETABLES

Yield: 4 servings
Dose per serving: black pepper 0.3 grams | cumin 0.8 grams |
fennel 0.4 grams | turmeric 0.5 grams

The delicious, nutty taste of dukkah pairs beautifully with olive oil and fresh vegetables.
Serve this simple roasted veggie dish with fresh bread or pita. You can even use it to top
a baked flatbread. Add some hummus and you're in spice heaven!

- 4 cups chopped vegetables (such as onions, zucchini, yellow squash, eggplant, peppers, or fennel bulb)
- 2 tablespoons olive oil
- 2 tablespoons Fennel Dukkah Blend

Adjust an oven rack to the middle position and preheat the oven to 400°F (200°C). Toss the vegetables with the olive oil and the Fennel Dukkah Blend and spread them in a single layer on a baking sheet. Bake for about 15 minutes, stirring occasionally, until the vegetables begin to brown at the edges (be careful not to let the Dukkah burn). Serve warm.

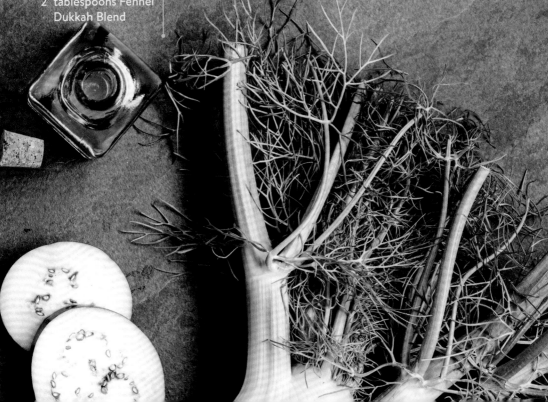

Heart Healthy Blend

Supports heart health, stabilizes blood sugar, acts as an anti-inflammatory

A delicious and powerful package perfect for cardiovascular support. If you prefer fresh garlic to dried, you can omit the garlic powder and add fresh garlic to taste just before using.

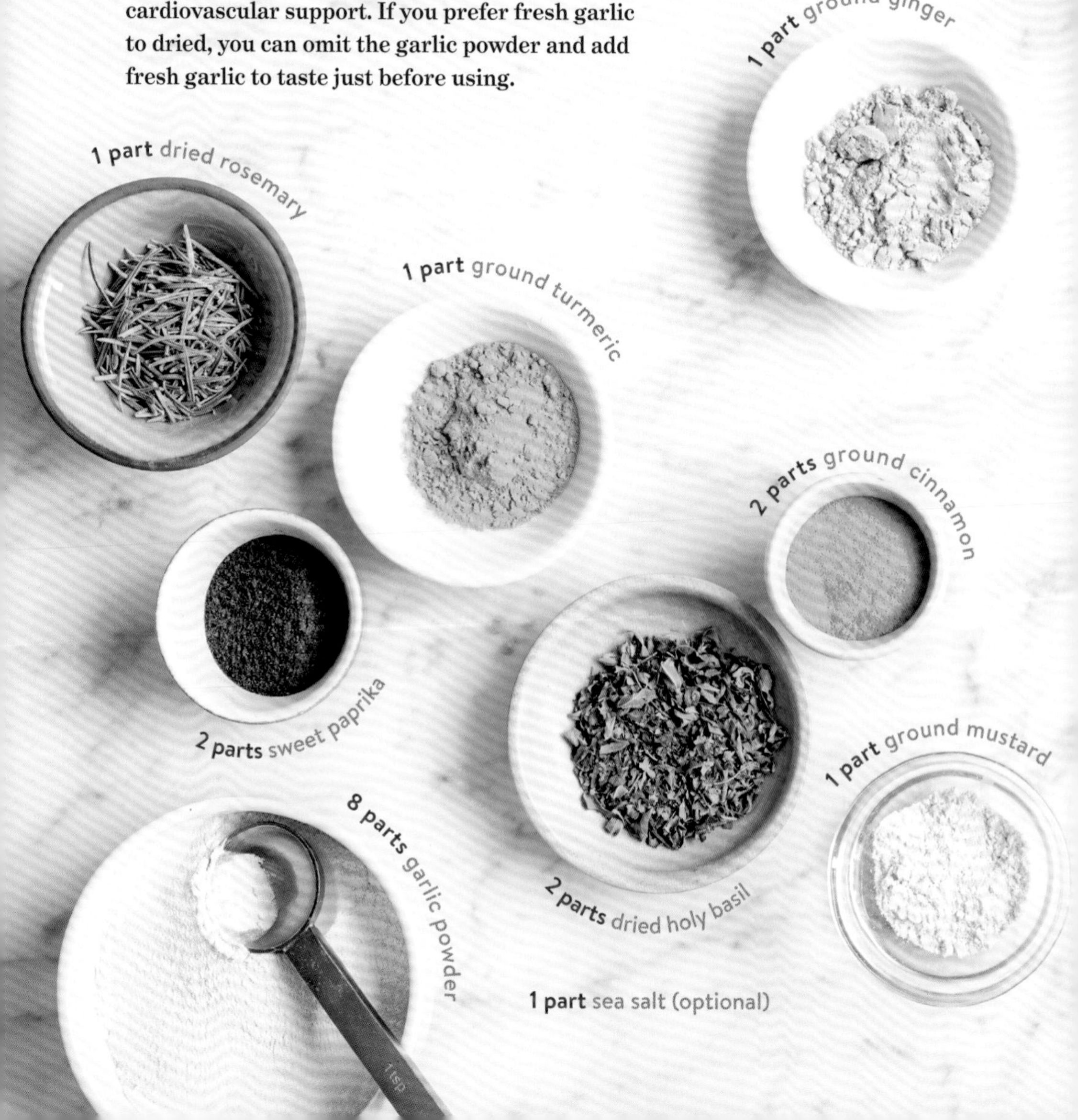

1 part ground ginger

1 part dried rosemary

1 part ground turmeric

2 parts ground cinnamon

2 parts sweet paprika

1 part ground mustard

8 parts garlic powder

2 parts dried holy basil

1 part sea salt (optional)

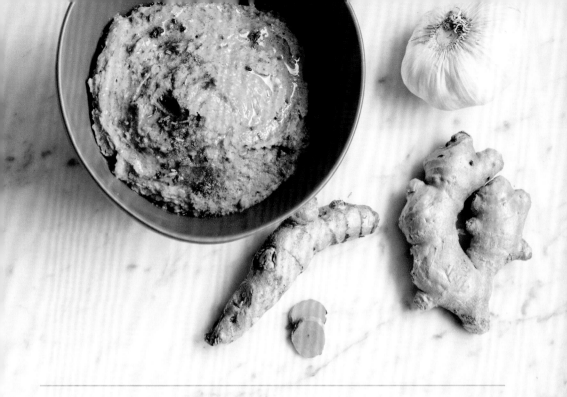

HEART HEALTHY HUMMUS

Yield: 1 serving

Dose per serving: cinnamon 0.9 grams | garlic 5.6 grams | ginger 0.5 grams | holy basil 0.3 grams | mustard 0.4 grams | rosemary 0.3 grams | turmeric 0.6 grams

Hummus is already a heart-healthy food. Adding a powerhouse medicinal spice blend to good-quality store-bought hummus is an easy way to make it even healthier — and more delicious. Serve with veggies, whole-grain bread, or crackers.

1 tablespoon Heart Healthy Blend

¼ cup of store-bought hummus

Olive oil for garnishing

Add the Heart Healthy Blend to hummus, stir it, and top with a drizzle of olive oil. Allow it to sit for at least an hour. Hummus will keep for about one week.

Cognitive Blend

Calms and nourishes, aids focus and memory, promotes mental alertness, acts as an anti-inflammatory, supports digestion

If you're experiencing mental fogginess or fatigue, this blend can help restore a calm, sharp mind. Add it to your cooking or sprinkle it over a finished dish. If you prefer the fresh versions of these herbs and spices, you can use those.

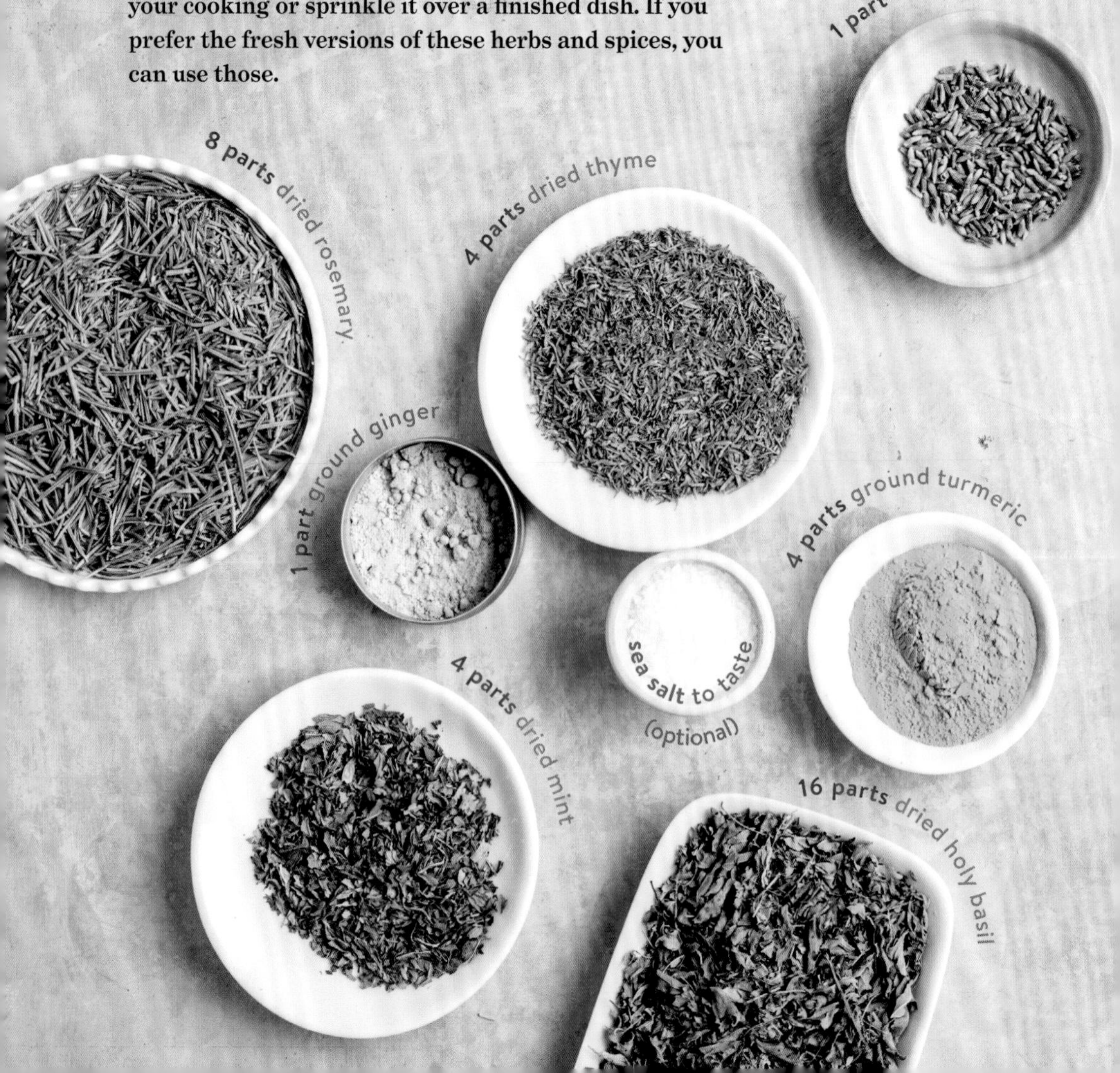

1 part dried lavender

8 parts dried rosemary

4 parts dried thyme

1 part ground ginger

4 parts ground turmeric

sea salt to taste (optional)

4 parts dried mint

16 parts dried holy basil

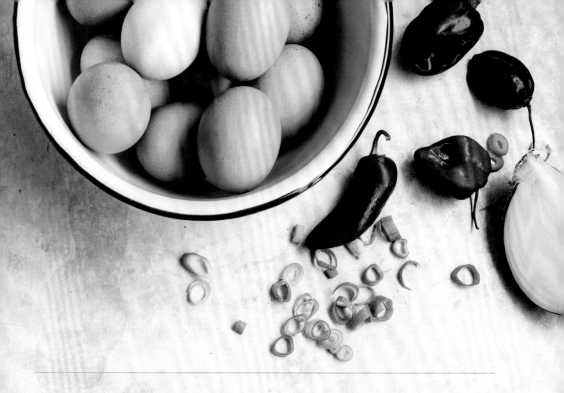

BOOMING BREAKFAST

Yield: 1 serving
Dose per serving: ginger 0.2 grams | holy basil 1.8 grams | lavender 0.1 grams |
mint 0.2 grams | rosemary 0.9 grams | thyme 0.3 grams | turmeric 0.7 grams

This easy spin on scrambled eggs or tofu will get your brain revved up and
ready to start the day right.

3 eggs or 8 ounces crumbled tofu

2 teaspoons Cognitive Blend

1 tablespoon butter

½ cup sautéed vegetables (such as peppers or onions)

¼ cup shredded cheddar cheese (optional)

Whisk the eggs with the Cognitive Blend until the mixture is uniform in color. Melt the butter in a large skillet over medium heat. Add the egg mixture and cook, stirring often, until large curds form. Add the sautéed vegetables and continue to cook until they begin to soften, about 1–2 minutes more. Off heat, sprinkle the cheese over the eggs and allow it to melt. Serve immediately.

Peppery Synergy Blend

Supports digestion, stabilizes blood sugar, acts as an anti-inflammatory, supports joint health, supports skin health

This spicy blend supports digestion and absorption of nutrients. It maximizes the benefits of turmeric because it contains black pepper to aid in the bioavailability of curcuminoids. You can make this blend as spicy as you want, but with black pepper present it will always have a bit of a kick!

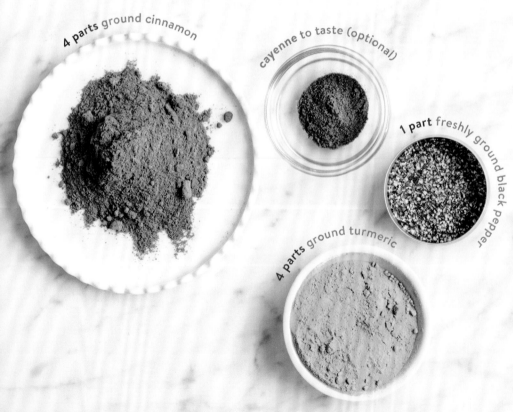

4 parts ground cinnamon

cayenne to taste (optional)

1 part freshly ground black pepper

4 parts ground turmeric

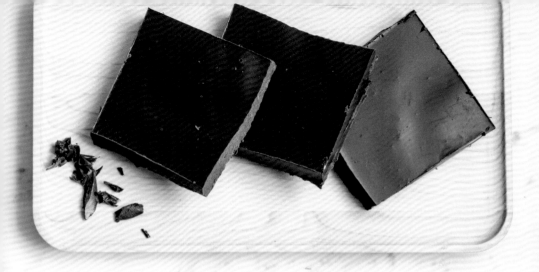

HEART SYNERGY FUDGE

Yield: 6 servings
Dose per serving: black pepper 0.46 grams | cinnamon 1.15 grams | turmeric 1.55 grams

This scrumptious but healthy fudge is an easy way to get a big dose of turmeric.
Unlike conventional fudge, which uses sugar as a stabilizer, this fudge will melt at
room temperature and is best stored in the fridge until ready to eat.

⅔ cup virgin
coconut oil

8 ounces dark
chocolate,
70-percent cacao,
chopped

2–4 tablespoons
Peppery Synergy
Blend

1 tablespoon
maple syrup
(optional)

1. In a double boiler or a heavy-bottomed saucepan, melt
   the oil over low heat. Add the chocolate and stir until
   completely melted. Stir in the Peppery Synergy Blend
   and the maple syrup, if using.

2. Pour the mixture into an 8-inch square glass baking
   dish and allow to cool slightly. When it has started to
   set, transfer to the refrigerator or freezer and let set
   completely, about 3 hours. Cut the fudge into pieces
   and serve cold.

Not Necessarily Spicy Chili Blend

Supports heart health, warms digestion, stabilizes blood sugar

This wonderful heart tonic uses medicine-packed mild chiles and is full of flavor, not heat. Add it right into your chili pot, or sprinkle it on tacos, fajitas, and grilled veggies. The mild and smoky-sweet flavor of ancho also lends itself well to hearty soups and stews, and can be used liberally.

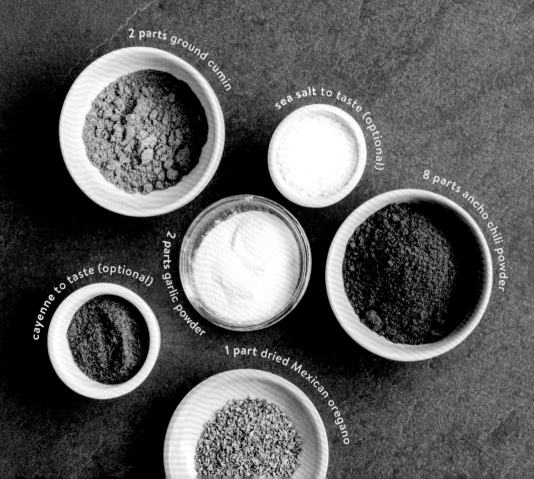

2 parts ground cumin

sea salt to taste (optional)

8 parts ancho chili powder

2 parts garlic powder

cayenne to taste (optional)

1 part dried Mexican oregano

RED CHILI POZOLE

Yield: 4 servings
Dose per serving: chile 14 grams | cumin 2.75 grams | garlic 3.8 grams

This traditional Mexican soup is made with hominy, which you can find in Latin American markets or in the international section of the grocery store. You can substitute chicken, ground beef, tofu, or ground tempeh for the steak, but it may require more or less cooking time in step 2. Feel free to use whatever type of broth or stock you have on hand — chicken, beef, or vegetable. Serve with arepas or cornbread.

3 tablespoons olive oil

1 cup diced onion

6 ounces steak, cut into bite-size pieces

½ cup Not Necessarily Spicy Chili Blend, plus more for seasoning

2 cups diced vegetables (such as tomatoes, carrots, corn, greens, zucchini, peppers, or scallions)

1 (15-ounce) can white hominy

4 cups broth or stock

Salt

Chili powder

1. Heat the oil in a large pot over medium heat. Add the onion and cook until it starts to soften, 2 to 3 minutes.

2. Add the steak and cook until it is cooked through, about 5 minutes. Stir in the Not Necessarily Spicy Chili Blend and cook until fragrant, 1 to 2 minutes.

3. Add the vegetables and cook until they begin to soften, 3 to 4 minutes. Add the hominy and the broth and simmer until the flavors meld, about 10 minutes more. Season with salt and additional chili powder to taste. Serve warm.

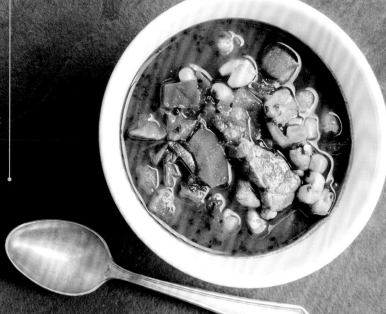

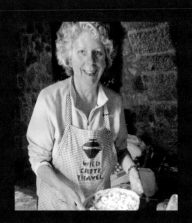

PATRICIA KYRITSI HOWELL is a Greek-American herbalist and cook who delights in using spices for flavor and healing. She is co-owner of Wild Crete Travel, a company specializing in small group tours that explore the traditional cuisine of the Greek island of Crete. Patricia points out that there isn't just one Greek cuisine, but that Greece has a variety of regional culinary influences. While regions in the north are influenced by Balkan culture, food on the Greek islands depends on each one's unique ecology. Islands in the eastern Aegean near the coast of Turkey have a Middle Eastern slant; while Crete has been at the crossroads of cultural influences for thousands of years.

Howell, whose great-grandmother was born on Crete, says the cuisine is diverse. The western part of the island is still influenced by Venetians who occupied the island from 1205 to 1571, and the eastern end of the island leans towards Turkish cuisine, as the island was once part of the Ottoman Empire. Though herbs and spices are used liberally, they tend to be milder flavors. "Greeks do not typically like strong spices or heat in their food," Patricia explains. "Greek cooking is very simple with an emphasis on high-quality, seasonal ingredients." She says Greeks do include aromatic Mediterranean herbs in most dishes, and they regard them as important for good digestion. Oregano is the most popular culinary herb and is usually not cooked but rather added to a dish after it's been served to preserve its aromatic qualities. In many restaurants, you'll find a shaker of oregano on the table next to the salt and pepper.

I asked Patricia about how people in Crete use herbs and spices for medicine and she explained that the most common usage is in teas or infusions (alcohol extracts or tinctures are not used). "Greeks believe that the aromatic quality of the tea is part of its healing properties, and we take great pleasure in savoring the fragrance." One common preparation is Mountain Tea. There is no standard recipe for this infusion. Each village has its own version, as do most families. It is made using the dried leaves and flowers of two plants native to Crete: malotira and dittany.

PATRICIA'S
GREEK HERBS AND SPICES
FOR FOOD AND MEDICINE

Malotira (*Sideritis syriaca*): This mint family herb grows at high elevations in the White Mountains of Crete and around the peak known as Psiloritis. The name malotira means "takes out what is bad." Malotira tastes like sage but is less harsh. It is considered a tonic, and many people drink it daily. It is also a specific for colds and respiratory congestion.

Dittany or Diktamos (*Origanum dictamnus*): The most important medicinal herb on Crete and in many parts of Greece. Until recently, it was only wild-harvested from high elevations in the mountains, where collecting it required braving steep and dangerous rock outcroppings. Now it is cultivated widely and is considered a panacea used for headaches, stomach pains, liver conditions, skin inflammation, and rashes. It has been part of Greek medicine since the time of Theophrastus, who recommended it as an aid to childbirth; it is said that Aphrodite used it to relieve labor pains. A tonic said to strengthen a weak constitution, it's also referred to as an erondas, a plant that restores youth.

Masticha (*Pistacia lentiscus*): The sun-dried resin of a tree that grows on the island of Chios, masticha was the original chewing gum used to freshen the breath and heal inflammation of the gums. It is made into liqueur and used to aid digestion and relieve cold symptoms. It has been studied for its ability to inhibit *H. pylori* bacteria, but it is also a popular flavoring for pastries and ice cream. The resin comes in small chunks known as tears, which are pounded in a mortar with a small amount of sugar and added to a recipe.

Sage (*Salvia trilobal*): Popular for tea, especially in cold and damp winter weather. It is commonly served at cafés near harbors or places frequented by fisherman and others who work on the water.

Oregano (*Origanum anites* and *O. vulgare*, ssp. *hirtum*): Commonly found in the wild on Crete and other parts of Greece, the flowering tops of both species are used — not just the leaf, as in the US. The most important spice in Greek cooking, it is added to salads, roasted meats, grilled fish, and the popular street food souvlaki (grilled chunks of chicken or pork). It is used in teas for respiratory congestion, stomach aches, and sometimes diarrhea. One folk tradition claims that women wash their breasts with oregano tea to keep them beautiful — but I know of no one doing this!

Rosemary (*Rosmarinus officinalis*): Mixed with red wine vinegar, olive oil, and garlic for meat marinades; it is also put on the fire when grilling meat to flavor the meat aromatically.

Basil (*Ocimum sanctum*): Rarely used in cooking, it is used ceremonially. Cultivated in pots and kept outside the doors of homes for good fortune. The leaves are also used during rituals in the Greek Orthodox Church to sprinkle holy water and be placed near sacred icons.

Thyme (*Thymus vulgaris*): Greek teas are often sweetened liberally with thyme honey, which is considered an important medicine used for coughs, colds, upset stomachs, and headaches. Thyme is a common wild herb, especially in coastal areas, and beekeepers often place their hives near stands of the plant.

Patricia's Masticha Ice Cream

One of Patricia's favorite recipes for ice cream is flavored with mastic resin. One taste sends me back to the island of Crete and all the delicious moments I had there!

½ cup sugar

½ teaspoon mastic resin

1 cup heavy cream

1 cup milk

4 egg yolks

1 tablespoon mastic liqueur (*optional*)

1. Grind the sugar and the mastic in a mortar and pestle. In a medium saucepan, heat the cream, the milk, and the sugar-mastic mixture over medium heat until it is almost boiling, about 5 minutes. Reduce heat to low.

2. In a medium bowl, whisk together the egg yolks. Whisking constantly, slowly pour in half of the cream mixture to temper the eggs. Stir the egg mixture back into the saucepan, along with the liqueur, if using. Cook until the mixture thickens and coats the back of a spoon. Strain through a fine-mesh strainer into a clean bowl.

3. Let the ice cream base chill in the fridge until it is completely cool. Churn according to your ice cream maker's instructions.

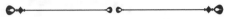

CURRIES

A curry can be any of a wide variety of dishes that use a combination of spices, including turmeric, cumin, coriander, ginger, and chiles. Originating on the Indian subcontinent, curry is generally prepared as a sauce mixed with meat and vegetables. There are many different, delicious curry spice blends from regions of India as well as Myanmar, Thailand, Malaysia, Vietnam, China, and Japan. Jamaica and other islands of the West Indies also commonly feature curries in their cuisines.

If you are beginning to experiment with curry, the good news is that there are lots of high-quality, tasty, and affordable premade curry blends out there. You can buy and try a few and then begin adding spices or recreating them at home. Indian curries tend to use lot of turmeric, cumin, and ginger.

Curries from Thailand make use of fresh, tangy herbs such as galangal and kaffir lime leaves. They frequently also contain fish sauce and might be combined with coconut milk. Massaman curry is the least spicy of the Thai varieties. The curries of Malaysia and Myanmar are a fusion of the Indian and Thai styles; curries that come from areas of Japan and China have a consistency similar to gravy. You can buy premixed curry blends as either powders or pastes at many grocery stores or specialty markets.

CARROT-ONION-TURMERIC CURRY

Sweet carrots and onions balance out pungent spices in this simple Indian-style curry packed with medicinal power. An extra dose of turmeric provides a beneficial boost. Mix this curry with any cooked meat, tofu, or other vegetables and serve over rice for a satisfying and crowd-pleasing dinner.

2 tablespoons olive oil	2 tablespoons curry powder	In a large skillet, heat the oil over medium heat. Add the onions and the carrots and cook until the vegetables begin to soften and brown, 5 to 7 minutes. Add the curry powder, garlic, and turmeric and stir to coat the vegetables. Continue cooking until the carrots are tender, about 5 minutes longer. Serve warm.
2 medium onions, cut into ½-inch pieces	2 cloves garlic, crushed	
4 carrots, peeled and cut into 2-inch pieces	½ teaspoon ground turmeric	

FRESH HERB AND SPICE RECIPES

Using fresh spices and herbs offers great flavor, and combining them with dried spices just increases their versatility. You can find good-quality fresh herbs and spices in many grocery stores, but growing them in your own garden or backyard pots is extra satisfying and helpful when creating simple daily dishes. Although fresh herbs and spices are more perishable than their dried counterparts, all of the recipes in this section can be stored for a few days in the fridge or frozen for about six weeks.

GARLIC SPREAD

Fresh garlic and olive oil — what's not to love? Full of garlicky goodness, this spread is great to use as a sauce, marinade, soup base, or anything else you want to embolden with aromatics.

½ cup olive oil, peanut oil, or untoasted sesame oil

1 head of garlic, peeled and crushed or finely chopped

1 fresh chile, seeded and chopped

1 tablespoon grated gingerroot

2 teaspoons grated fresh turmeric or ½ teaspoon ground turmeric

1 teaspoon dried holy basil

½ teaspoon ground mustard

Salt

Stir together the oil, garlic, chile, ginger, turmeric, holy basil, and mustard and mix until smooth. Season with salt to taste and serve (or store in the refrigerator for up to one month).

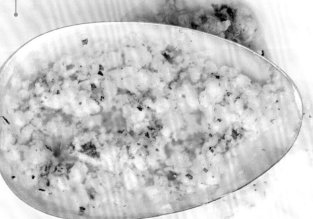

MEDICINAL MISO SOUP

Miso is a traditional Japanese flavoring made from fermented soybeans, salt, koji spores, and often barley. Some misos are mild and sweet, while others are aged and tangy; shop around to find one you like. Adding Garlic Spread to this healthy soup base gives it a full-bodied medicinal kick. No cooking required! It's perfect to bring to work as a salty, savory afternoon pick-me-up.

1 cup miso paste

2 tablespoons Garlic Spread

½ teaspoon ground mustard (optional)

In a small bowl, stir together miso, Garlic Spread, and mustard powder, if using, until well combined. Store in the refrigerator for up to four days.

To use: Mix 2 tablespoons Medicinal Miso Soup mix with 16 ounces hot water.

PESTO POWER!

This well-known and well-loved herb sauce is traditionally made with basil, pine nuts, olive oil, garlic, salt, and Parmesan cheese. But we don't have to stick to tradition with pesto; there are hundreds of variations. Garlic often makes an appearance but isn't strictly necessary. Pesto can be made with nearly all aromatic leaves, sometimes in combination with non-aromatic leaves or greens to provide more nutrition. The combination of leafy herbs, oil, nuts, and salt is such a good one I find myself rummaging around in the garden or the produce drawer for whatever I can throw into the food processor.

THE BEST FOR PESTO

Primary fresh greens: mint, parsley, lemon balm, skullcap, basil, holy basil, bee balm, arugula, watercress, nasturtium, nettles, spinach, kale

Additional fresh herbs: fennel, sage, cilantro, rosemary, thyme, dill, goldenrod leaves

Oils: olive, avocado, grapeseed, almond, sunflower, walnut, hazelnut, sesame (untoasted)

Nuts and seeds: pine nuts, pistachios, hazelnuts, macadamia nuts, sesame seeds, sunflower seeds

Extras: garlic, lemon peel, lemon juice, salt

MINDFUL PESTO

This tasty, semi-traditional pesto with holy basil has brain-nourishing rosemary as well as walnuts and walnut oil to maximize its cognition-enhancing potential. Spread it on crackers, add it to pasta dishes, and use it as a marinade.

2 cups fresh holy basil leaves

½ cup walnut oil or olive oil

½ cup walnuts or pine nuts

8 cloves garlic

2 tablespoons fresh rosemary, finely chopped

1 tablespoon fresh lemon juice

Salt

Process the basil, oil, walnuts, garlic, rosemary, and lemon juice in a food processor until smooth. (Alternatively, you can chop everything by hand or use a mortar and pestle, though the texture will be coarser.) Season with salt to taste. Store in small portions in the freezer for up to nine months.

EAT YOUR GREENS PESTO

Loaded with leafy greens, this pesto is perfect for everyday use. You can use arugula, watercress, spinach, kale, or nettle leaves — my favorite is a blend of nettles and arugula. Whether stirred into pasta, smothered on bread, or served with meat, fish, or tofu, you can't go wrong with this all-purpose sauce.

3 cups leafy greens

1 cup olive oil

1 cup fresh basil leaves

½ cup pine nuts

4 cloves garlic

1 ounce Parmesan cheese, grated (optional)

Salt

Process the greens, oil, basil, pine nuts, garlic, and cheese, if using, in a food processor until smooth. Season with salt to taste. Store in small portions in the freezer for up to three months (note that if using cheese, the texture may suffer after freezing).

PARSLEY PESTO

This spin on pesto is not only delicious but also supports healthy kidneys, urinary function, and prostate health. Parsley is widely available and has a longer growing season than basil, so it's a great choice for pesto. Pistachios can be time-consuming to shell but, I think, are absolutely worth the effort.

2 cups fresh parsley leaves

½ cup pistachios, shelled

½ cup olive oil

1 teaspoon lemon zest

½ teaspoon celery seed

Salt

Fresh lemon juice

Process the parsley, pistachios, oil, lemon zest, and celery seed in a food processor until well-ground but not smooth. (Alternatively, you can chop everything by hand or use a mortar and pestle, though the texture will be coarser.) Season with salt and lemon juice to taste.

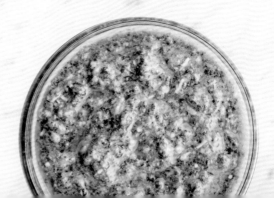

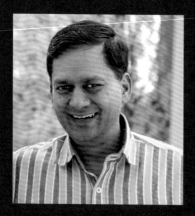

SANDEEP AGARWAL is the fifth-generation owner of Pure Generation Foods, a manufacturer of spices, ghee, and other Ayurvedic products. He is also an herbalist who brings a wealth of knowledge to the table regarding herbal medicine.

"You can't imagine Indian foods without herbs and spices," says Sandeep. "Indian food uses many spices, but that doesn't mean that it is spicy. It simply means it is flavorful." Curry might be the first dish we think of, but the term doesn't refer to a single specific blend of spices or one recipe. Sandeep explains that Indian curries are made by sautéing fresh onion, garlic, ginger, and chile — with other fresh herbs and dried spices — in ghee or oil. Thousands of combinations of herbs and spices can make up a curry blend.

More than 40 different spices are typically used in Indian cuisine, the most common ones being black pepper, cardamom, chile, cinnamon, clove, coriander, cumin, turmeric, fennel, ginger, garlic, mustard seeds, and fenugreek. Blends can be sweet, spicy, or all-out searing. Heating spices and herbs with fats allows the medicinal value to become bioavailable; and while making

is filled with a lovely aroma that kicks off digestion. The sauce is then combined with vegetables, grains, or meats to make the final dish.

SPICES FOR HEALING

Medicinal spices are often used in very simple ways in India. For example, chewing a slice of fresh ginger with a pinch of salt before a meal stokes the digestive fire. Or a pinch of clove mixed with a teaspoon of honey is very effective for treating a cough. And for cold, flu, or fever, Sandeep might use holy basil.

We might not think of milk as a base for medicine, but Sandeep says many medicinal spice preparations are made with a base of warm milk: "Every Indian mother knows that warm milk with turmeric and ghee is great for the common cold." Another medicinal use of turmeric is for small cuts and bruises, where a pinch of turmeric mixed with warm ghee is applied topically. Warm milk is also prepared with saffron, cardamom, and ghee as an aphrodisiac. "A new bride traditionally offers this drink to her spouse on their first night together," Sandeep says.

Triphala, literally translated as "three fruits," is a traditional Ayurvedic formulation made from three native Indian fruits: amalaki (*Emblica officinalis*), bibhitaki (*Terminalia bellirica*), and haritaki (*Terminalia chebula*). People use this as a daily tonic, taking a half-teaspoon with warm water before bed for healthy digestion and gentle everyday detoxification. Sandeep says Triphala is called the "nectar of life" for its cleansing, balancing, and healing properties.

Sandeep's Kitchari

Kitchari is a delicious stew of basmati rice and husked split mung beans. It is cooked like oatmeal along with salt and Indian spices. It is easy to digest and is traditionally consumed when someone is sick or recovering from an illness.

3½ cups water

1 cup assorted vegetables (optional)

½ cup basmati rice

½ cup mung dal (split yellow dried)

½ teaspoon cumin seed (whole or powder)

½ teaspoon coriander powder

½ teaspoon mustard seed (whole or powder)

½ teaspoon turmeric powder

1 teaspoon ginger-root, chopped or grated

½ teaspoon salt

3 teaspoons grass-fed organic ghee

1 handful fresh cilantro leaves

Remove any foreign substances such as small stones or soil particles from the rice and mung dal, and then rinse with water. In a stockpot, add the water, vegetables, rice, mung dal, cumin, coriander, mustard seed, turmeric, ginger, and salt. Bring the mixture to a boil, then reduce heat to low and partially cover. Simmer, stirring occasionally, for 20 minutes, or until it reaches the consistency of a stew. Add more water if needed. Once done, remove from heat and add ghee. Mix well. Garnish with cilantro leaves and serve hot.

INSTANT LEMON-GINGER HERBAL TEA

Use this mix to make instant hot or iced tea to ward off colds and flu, support healthy digestion, and decrease inflammation.

2 tablespoons honey or maple syrup

½ tablespoon lemon zest plus 2 table-spoons lemon juice

1 tablespoon grated gingerroot

1 teaspoon ground turmeric

To use: Add 1 teaspoon Instant Lemon-Ginger Herbal Tea mix to 8 ounces of hot or cold water and let steep until desired flavor is achieved.

HOT GINGER LEMONADE

This is a great winter beverage, especially during the holiday season when friends, family, and germs all come together to mix and mingle.

1 (4-inch) piece of fresh gingerroot, peeled and thinly sliced

2 lemons, each cut into 4 wedges

Cloves (optional)

Honey

1. In a large saucepan, add the ginger to 8 cups of water and bring to a boil. Reduce the heat to medium low, cover, and simmer for 20 minutes.

2. To serve, stick a few cloves, if using, into the rind of each lemon wedge. Squeeze the juice from each wedge into a mug, then drop the wedge in. Pour 8 ounces of the ginger-infused water into each mug. Add honey to taste.

Note: You can keep the ginger water on low heat, adding fresh water as needed, for several hours.

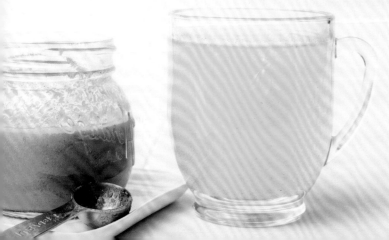

APPENDIX: A HEALTHCARE PRACTITIONER'S GUIDE TO USING MEDICINAL SPICES

If you are a healthcare provider interested in integrative medicine and nutrition, you may have encountered information about the medicinal use of herbs and spices. Many of these are the same culinary spices used widely in cuisines across the world. However, without specific and consistent medicinal dosage information it can be challenging to recommend using spices to clients.

It is my goal to offer some information you can use to translate health outcomes research into practical client-care strategies. Often, the simplest solutions are also the most effective and the most practical. If a client can introduce small amounts of spices in her food regularly, expensive supplements and complicated products are not necessary. Spices are generally less expensive than commercial healthcare products, which is especially beneficial when working with low-income or underserved communities. Additionally, when consumed as food, spices are more bioavailable and reap synergistic benefits compared to extracts and supplements.

GUIDELINES FOR RECOMMENDING SPICES TO CLIENTS

When you walk the path of natural medicine and move out of a pharmaceutical-based approach to health, you find yourself in a place where things are a more organic, more sensory, and also bit more ambiguous. The precise and prescribed dosage of a pill can feel reassuring, but as you learn about using spices as medicine you'll find that precision in dosing is not especially important regarding safety as well as outcomes. What is important when using spices as dietary medicine is consistency of usage, sustainability of the practice, and understanding bioavailability. Regarding consistency of usage, research shows that consuming a medicinal spice regularly — not on a strict schedule or precise dosage — can have beneficial effects.

INTRODUCING NEW HABITS

When evaluating a client, it is best to begin with an understanding of her current dietary habits. If the client identifies with a particular cultural or geographic cuisine that uses specific spices, this can be a great place to start thinking about which spices to focus on. You can find a list of some of the most commonly used spices in specific regions around the world on page 112. Asking a client about her favorite spice or groups of spices can also be a good place to start. If a client generally likes flavorful foods, you have many opportunities to introduce new spices. If you are working with someone who prefers a bland diet or consumes a lot of processed foods, you may need to take baby steps with small amounts of spices. This type of client might start with adding spice blends to a dish once it has been cooked (see the recipes for spice blends beginning on page 116). It can also be good to start with spices that are fairly common and well-known, such as garlic, ginger, cinnamon, mint, or black pepper, as the client's palate adjusts. Also, be sure to ask which spices may already be part of a client's diet. Clients might be currently consuming and enjoying a beneficial spice but only in limited doses. In this case, your suggestions can be simple modifications to increase consumption.

DOSAGE

Choosing a dose to recommend is probably the most complicated aspect of prescribing medicinal spices. One initial approach is to ask the client to simply integrate the spice into her diet on a daily basis at whatever dose she can. This may be the easiest way for you and the client to see if the spice is a good fit. However, it doesn't ensure that the client will be getting enough of the spice for optimal health outcomes. Daily dose recommendations for each spice are given in both grams and dietary teaspoon equivalents in chapter 3. These are suggestions for one spice and its specific therapeutic value. If several spices are combined, they benefit from a synergistic effect, and dosages can be reduced. Recommending a dose in grams per day, or the teaspoon equivalent, added to food preparation will give clients a measurable goal. One easy way to assure compliance and correct dosage is to recommend that a client make a week's or month's

quantity of one spice blend and divide it into daily portions. The recipes in this book offer a starting place for clients to begin integrating a specific spice into their diets every day — especially a spice they likely have not already been using regularly. In addition, there are, of course, hundreds of cookbooks and recipe websites you can recommend for clients who are looking to expand their practice of integrating spices into their cuisine.

ACCESSIBLE, AFFORDABLE, PREVENTIVE MEDICINE

Spices offer a good option for preventive medicines that are affordable, relatively familiar, and easy to incorporate into daily life. They can be used to treat the whole family.

HEALTHY FAMILIES

One of my favorite ways to use medicinal spices is feeding families as a whole. Considering the social determinants of health, some children are more at risk of developing specific health conditions such as heart disease or diabetes. The spices in this book are used for prevention and treatment of the most common conditions that affect underserved or marginalized populations, including diabetes, heart disease, arthritis, joint conditions, infections, and immune concerns. As a healthcare practitioner you have an opportunity to administer medicinal spices to the entire family for both treatment and prevention. When spices are included in family meals, adults receive the medicine they need for specific conditions, while younger family members are helping to prevent early stages of conditions and are learning to enjoy the flavors and integrate this wellness practice into their lives.

AFFORDABILITY AND ACCESS

Some spices are expensive or difficult to acquire, such as cardamom and vanilla. Fortunately, many of our most medicinal spices are readily available and affordable, including garlic, ginger, turmeric, cumin, and cinnamon. Additionally, these spices are shelf stable.

The brand name spice jars on supermarket shelves are the most expensive way to buy a spice. I advise clients to buy in bulk. Many Asian, Indian, and Latin American grocery stores stock spices in larger bags that are affordable and contain enough for several weeks' worth of family meals. Health food stores often carry spices in bulk bins, and you can purchase any quantity you want by weight. When clients get home, they should ideally transfer the spices into glass jars; clean pasta sauce jars work well. Plastic bags also are good options. I prefer glass jars if they can be kept somewhere

dark, but jars can be impractical if you don't have the shelf space.

If your client population has access to a garden, community garden plot, or even a potted garden, there are many possibilities for cultivating spices. Depending on the geographic region, spices such as rosemary, thyme, sage, chives, and parsley can be grown easily. These fresh herbs have long lifetimes once planted, and they offer plenty of medicine for minimal expense. Fresh spices can be used liberally and offer significant health benefits.

Finally, spice blends can be ideal for clients who have limited financial means, as they can be easily added to cooking. As a practitioner, you could order a quantity of common spices and create some of the spice blend recipes from this book to distribute to clients. Alternately, you can provide recipes to clients, and they can blend the spices according to their own preferences.

Regardless of your approach, the idea is to make it easy, pleasurable, and affordable for your clients to access and enjoy medicinal spices. Used thoughtfully, this delicious medicine will become an enjoyable part of their lives.

ACKNOWLEDGMENTS

With each click of the key in writing this book, I felt thankful for the many hands and hearts who harvested and processed the spices I have access to and for the millions of plants that create such masterpieces of nature. I'm thankful to Anne Harvey and Kristen McPhee for their countless hours helping me find and evaluate research for this book, and for Camille Freeman for being the person I could always bounce an idea (or twelve) off of. Carleen Madigan, my editor, was always there willing to listen and provide as many answers as I had questions. A huge thanks to Patricia Kyritsi Howell, Michael Tims, Sandeep Agarwal, Funke Kolosheo, the folks at the Tangawizi Spice Farm, and Jennifer Gerrity and Mountain Rose for sharing their time and expertise with me — it really allowed me to paint a more global picture of spices, and for that I am grateful! Thanks to Maria Noël Groves and Rosalee de la Forêt for helping me negotiate the logistics of being a first-time book author. And thanks to my family, who gave up time with me so I could tap away at my computer wherever we were around the globe.

BIBLIOGRAPHY

BLACK PEPPER

Abullais, S. S., Dani, N., Hamiduddin, N. P., Kudyar, N., and Gore, A. (2015). Efficacy of irrigation with different antimicrobial agents on periodontal health in patients treated for chronic periodontitis: A randomized controlled clinical trial. *Ayu*, 36(4), 380.

Pipalia, P. R., Annigeri, R. G., and Mehta, R. (2016). Clinicobiochemical evaluation of turmeric with black pepper and *Nigella sativa* in management of oral submucous fibrosis — a double-blind, randomized preliminary study. Oral Surgery, Oral Medicine, Oral Pathology and Oral Radiology, 122(6), 705–712.

Srinivasan, K. (2007). Black pepper and its pungent principle — piperine: a review of diverse physiological effects. *Critical Reviews in Food Science and Nutrition*, 47(8), 735–748.

CALENDULA

Carvalho, A. F. M. D., Feitosa, M. C. P., Coelho, N. P. M. D. F., Rebêlo, V. C. N., Castro, J. G. D., Sousa, P. R. G. D., . . . and Arisawa, E. A. L. S. (2016). Low-level laser therapy and *Calendula officinalis* in repairing diabetic foot ulcers. *Revista da Escola de Enfermagem da USP*, 50(4), 628–634.

Duran, V., Matic, M., Jovanović, M., Mimica, N., Gajinov, Z., Poljack, M., and Boza, P. (2005). Results of the clinical examination of an ointment with marigold (*Calendula officinalis*) extract in the treatment of venous leg ulcers. *Int J Tissue React.* 27(3),101–6.

Panahi, Y., Sharif, M. R., Sharif, A., Beiraghdar, F., Zahiri, Z., Amirchoopani, G., . . . and Sahebkar, A. (2012). A randomized comparative trial on the therapeutic efficacy of topical aloe vera and *Calendula officinalis* on diaper dermatitis in children. *The Scientific World Journal*, 2012.

CHILE PEPPER

Ertürk, Ö. (2006). Antibacterial and antifungal activity of ethanolic extracts from eleven spice plants. Biologia, Bratislava, 61/3: 275–278, 2006. *Cellular and Molecular Biology.*

Janssens, P. L., Hursel, R., and Westerterp-Plantenga, M. S. (2014). Capsaicin increases sensation of fullness in energy balance, and decreases desire to eat after dinner in negative energy balance. *Appetite*, 77, 46–51.

CINNAMON

Akilen, R., Tsiami, A., Devendra, D., and Robinson, N. (2010). Glycated haemoglobin and blood pressure lowering effect of cinnamon in multi ethnic Type 2 diabetic patients in the UK: a randomized, placebo controlled, double blind clinical trial. *Diabetic Medicine*, 27(10), 1159–1167.

Khan, A., Safdar, M., Khan, M. M. A., Khattak, K. N., and Anderson, R. A. (2003). Cinnamon improves glucose and lipids of people with type 2 diabetes. *Diabetes Care*, 26(12), 3215–3218.

Shishehbor, F., Rezaeyan Safar, M., Rajaei, E., and Haghighizadeh, M. H. (2018). Cinnamon Consumption Improves Clinical Symptoms and Inflammatory Markers in Women With Rheumatoid Arthritis. *Journal of the American College of Nutrition*, 1–6.

CUMIN

Taghizadeh, M., Memarzadeh, M. R., Asemi, Z., and Esmaillzadeh, A. (2015). Effect of the cumin cyminum L. intake on weight loss, metabolic profiles and biomarkers of oxidative stress in overweight subjects: a randomized double-blind placebo-controlled clinical trial. *Annals of Nutrition and Metabolism*, 66(2–3), 117–124.

FENNEL

Portincasa, P., Bonfrate, L., Scribano, M. L., Kohn, A., Caporaso, N., Festi, D., . . . and Fogli, M. V. (2016). Curcumin and Fennel Essential Oil Improve Symptoms and Quality of Life in Patients with Irritable Bowel Syndrome. *Journal of Gastrointestinal and Liver Diseases*, 25(2).

GARLIC

Arreola, R., Quintero-Fabián, S., López-Roa, R. I., Flores-Gutiérrez, E. O., Reyes-Grajeda, J. P., Carrera-Quintanar, L., and Ortuño-Sahagún, D. (2015). Immunomodulation and anti-inflammatory effects of garlic compounds. *Journal of Immunology Research*, 2015.

Budoff, M. J., Ahmadi, N., Gul, K. M., Liu, S. T., Flores, F. R., Tiano, J., . . . and Tsimikas, S. (2009). Aged garlic extract supplemented with B vitamins, folic acid and L-arginine retards the progression of subclinical atherosclerosis: a randomized clinical trial. *Preventive Medicine*, 49(2–3), 101–107.

Jain, A. K., Vargas, R., Gotzkowsky, S., and McMahon, F. G. (1993). Can garlic reduce levels of serum lipids? A controlled clinical study. *The American Journal of Medicine*, 94(6), 632–635.

Josling, P. (2001). Preventing the common cold with a garlic supplement: a double-blind, placebo-controlled survey. *Advances in Therapy*, 18(4), 189–193.

Sivam, G. P. (2001). Protection against *Helicobacter pylori* and other bacterial infections by garlic. *The Journal of Nutrition*, 131(3), 1106S–1108S.

Stevinson, C., Pittler, M. H., and Ernst, E. (2000). Garlic for treating hypercholesterolemia: a meta-analysis of randomized clinical trials. *Annals of Internal Medicine*, 133(6), 420–429.

Warshafsky, S., Kamer, R. S., and Sivak, S. L. (1993). Effect of garlic on total serum cholesterol: a meta-analysis. *Annals of Internal Medicine*, 119(7_Part_1), 599–605.

GINGER

Akoachere, J. T., Ndip, R. N., Chenwi, E. B., Ndip, L. M., Njock, T. E., and Anong, D. N. (2002). Antibacterial effects of *Zingiber Officinale* and *Garcinia Kola* on respiratory tract pathogens. *East African Medical Journal*, 79(11), 588–592.

Black, C. D., Herring, M. P., Hurley, D. J., and O'Connor, P. J. (2010). Ginger (*Zingiber officinale*) reduces muscle pain caused by eccentric exercise. *The Journal of Pain*, 11(9), 894–903.

Boone, S. A., and Shields, K. M. (2005). Treating pregnancy-related nausea and vomiting with ginger. *Annals of Pharmacotherapy*, 39(10), 1710–1713.

Kulkarni, R. A., and Deshpande, A. R. (2016). Anti-inflammatory and antioxidant effect of ginger in tuberculosis. *Journal of Complementary and Integrative Medicine*, 13(2), 201–206.

Mashhadi, N., Ghasvand, R., Askari, G., Feizi, A., Hairiri, M., Darvishi, L., Bahrain, A., Taghiyr, M., Shiranian, A., and Hajishafiee, M. (2013). Influence of ginger and cinnamon intake on inflammation and muscle soreness endued by exercise in Iranian female athletes. *Int J Prev Med*. 2013 Apr; 4(Suppl 1): S11–S15.

Matsumura, M. D., Zavorsky, G. S., and Smoliga, J. M. (2015). The Effects of Pre Exercise Ginger Supplementation on Muscle Damage and Delayed Onset Muscle Soreness. *Phytotherapy Research*, 29(6), 887–893.

Mozaffari-Khosravi, H., Naderi, Z., Dehghan, A., Nadjarzadeh, A., and Fallah Huseini, H. (2016). Effect of Ginger Supplementation on Proinflammatory Cytokines in Older Patients with Osteoarthritis: Outcomes of a Randomized Controlled Clinical Trial. *Journal of Nutrition in Gerontology and Geriatrics*, 35(3), 209–218.

Prasad, S., and Tyagi, A. K. (2015). Ginger and its constituents: role in prevention and treatment of gastrointestinal cancer. *Gastroenterology Research and Practice*, 2015.

Saenghong, N., Wattanathorn, J., Muchimapura, S., Tongun, T., Piyavhatkul, N., Banchonglikitkul, C., and Kajsongkram, T. (2012). *Zingiber officinale* improves cognitive function of the middle-aged healthy woman. *Evidence-Based Complementary and Alternative Medicine*, 2012.

Srinivasan, K. (2014). Antioxidant potential of spices and their active constituents. *Critical Reviews in Food Science and Nutrition*, 54(3), 352–372.

Yusha'u, M., Garba, L., and Shamsuddeen, U. (2008). In vitro inhibitory activity of garlic and ginger extracts on some respiratory tract isolates of gram-negative organisms. *International Journal of Biomedical and Health Sciences*, 4(2).

HOLY BASIL

Bhattacharyya, D., Sur, T. K., Jana, U., and Debnath, P. K. (2008). Controlled programmed trial of *Ocimum sanctum* leaf on generalized anxiety disorders. *Nepal Med Coll J*, 10(3), 176–179.

Sampath, S., Mahapatra, S. C., Padhi, M. M., Sharma, R., and Talwar, A. (2015). Holy basil (*Ocimum sanctum Linn.*) leaf extract enhances specific cognitive parameters in healthy adult volunteers: A placebo controlled study. *Indian Journal of Physiology and Pharmacology*, 59(1), 69–77.

LAVENDER

Kao, Y. H., Huang, Y. C., Chung, U. L., Hsu, W. N., Tang, Y. T., and Liao, Y. H. (2017). Comparisons for Effectiveness of Aromatherapy and Acupressure Massage on Quality of Life in Career Women: A Randomized Controlled Trial. *The Journal of Alternative and Complementary Medicine*, 23(6), 451–460.

Lillehei, A. S., Halcón, L. L., Savik, K., and Reis, R. (2015). Effect of inhaled lavender and sleep hygiene on self-reported sleep issues: a randomized controlled trial. *The Journal of Alternative and Complementary Medicine*, 21(7), 430–438.

MINT

Cappello, G., Spezzaferro, M., Grossi, L., Manzoli, L., and Marzio, L. (2007). Peppermint oil (Mintoil®) in the treatment of irritable bowel syndrome: a prospective double blind placebo-controlled randomized trial. *Digestive and Liver Disease*, 39(6), 530–536.

MUSTARD

Gregersen, N. T., Belza, A., Jensen, M. G., Ritz, C., Bitz, C., Hels, O., . . . and Astrup, A. (2013). Acute effects of mustard, horseradish, black pepper and ginger on energy expenditure, appetite, ad libitum energy intake and energy balance in human subjects. *British Journal of Nutrition*, 109(3), 556–563.

Lett, A. M., Thondre, P. S., and Rosenthal, A. J. (2013). Yellow mustard bran attenuates glycaemic response of a semi-solid food in young healthy men. *International Journal of Food Sciences and Nutrition*, 64(2), 140–146.

ROSEMARY

Moss, M., Cook, J., Wesnes, K., and Duckett, P. (2003). Aromas of rosemary and lavender essential oils differentially affect cognition and mood in healthy adults. *International Journal of Neuroscience*, 113(1), 15–38.

Pengelly, A., Snow, J., Mills, S. Y., Scholey, A., Wesnes, K., and Butler, L. R. (2012). Short-term study on the effects of rosemary on cognitive function in an elderly population. *Journal of Medicinal Food*, 15(1), 10–17.

SAGE

Bommer, S., Klein, P., and Suter, A. (2011). First time proof of sage's tolerability and efficacy in menopausal women with hot flushes. *Advances in Therapy*, 28(6), 490–500.

Vandecasteele, K., Ost, P., Oosterlinck, W., Fonteyne, V., De Neve, W., and De Meerleer, G. (2012). Evaluation of the efficacy and safety of *Salvia officinalis* in controlling hot flashes in prostate cancer patients treated with androgen deprivation. *Phytotherapy Research*, 26(2), 208–213.

THYME

Kemmerich, B., Eberhardt, R., and Stammer, H. (2006). Efficacy and tolerability of a fluid extract combination of thyme herb and ivy leaves and matched placebo in adults suffering from acute bronchitis with productive cough. *Arzneimittelforschung*, 56(09), 652–660.

TURMERIC

Chuengsamarn, S., Rattanamongkolgul, S., Luechapudiporn, R., Phisalaphong, C., and Jirawatnotai, S. (2012). Curcumin extract for prevention of type 2 diabetes. *Diabetes Care*, 35(11), 2121–2127.

Gupta, S. C., Sung, B., Kim, J. H., Prasad, S., Li, S., and Aggarwal, B. B. (2013). Multitargeting by turmeric, the golden spice: from kitchen to clinic. *Molecular Nutrition and Food Research*, 57(9), 1510–1528.

Soni, K. B., and Kuttan, R. (1992). Effect of oral curcumin administration on serum peroxides and cholesterol levels in human volunteers. *Indian Journal of Physiology and Pharmacology*, 36, 273–273.

Thangapazham, R. L., Sharma, A., and Maheshwari, R. K. (2007). Beneficial role of curcumin in skin diseases. In *The Molecular Targets and Therapeutic Uses of Curcumin in Health and Disease* (pp. 343–357). Springer.

RESOURCES

To purchase quality spices in bulk, these companies offer affordability, reliability, and unique spice blends:

FRONTIER CO-OP

WWW.FRONTIERCOOP.COM

MOUNTAIN ROSE HERBS

WWW.MOUNTAINROSEHERBS.COM

OAKTOWN SPICE SHOP

HTTPS://OAKTOWNSPICESHOP.COM

PENZEYS

WWW.PENZEYS.COM

METRIC
CONVERSION CHART

WEIGHT		
TO CONVERT	TO	MULTIPLY
ounces	grams	ounces by 28.35
pounds	grams	pounds by 453.5
pounds	kilograms	pounds by 0.45

US	METRIC
0.035 ounce	1 gram
¼ ounce	7 grams
½ ounce	14 grams
1 ounce	28 grams
1½ ounces	40 grams
3½ ounces	100 grams
4 ounces	112 grams
8 ounces	228 grams
16 ounces (1 pound)	454 grams

Note: Unless you have finely calibrated measuring equipment, conversions between US and metric measurements will be somewhat inexact. It's important to convert the measurements for all of the ingredients in a recipe to maintain the same proportions as the original.

WEIGHT
CONVERSION CHART

MEDICINAL SPICE	EQUIVALENT WEIGHT (GRAMS TO ONE TSP)	EQUIVALENT WEIGHT (GRAMS TO ONE TBSP)
BLACK PEPPER	4.2g pwd	12.6g pwd
CALENDULA	0.5g petals	1.5g petals
CARDAMON	3.5g pwd	10.5g pwd
CELERY SEED	3g seed	9g seed
CHILES	3.8g pwd	11.5g pwd
CINNAMON	2.6g pwd	8g pwd
CUMIN	3g pwd or seed	9g pwd or seed
FENNEL	3.1g seed	9.3g seed
GARLIC	4.2g pwd	12.6g pwd
GINGER	3g pwd	9g pwd
HOLY BASIL	0.8g c/s	2.4g c/s
LAVENDER	1g flowers	3g flowers
MINT	1.1g c/s	3.3g c/s
MUSTARD	2.6g pwd or seed	7.8g pwd or seed
PARSLEY	0.7g c/s	2.3g c/s
ROSEMARY	2g c/s	6g c/s
SAGE	1.1g c/s	3.3g c/s
THYME	1.3g c/s	3.9g c/s
TURMERIC	3.5g pwd	10.5g pwd

INDEX

Page numbers in *italic* indicate images; numbers in **bold** indicate charts and tables.

I

IBS. *See* irritable bowel syndrome
Ice Cream, Patricia's Masticha, 144
immune protection and defense, 84–87,
    106–107
in vitro studies, 25
India, 112, 150–151
infections, **106–107**. *See also* immune
    protection and defense
inflammation, 22, 77, 105, **106–107**
Instant Lemon-Ginger Herbal Tea, 152
irritable bowel syndrome (IBS), 93, 96–97
isoflavones, 20
isothiocyanates, 87

J

Jamaica nutmeg (*Monodora myristica*),
    42–43
Jellies, Cinnamon Spice, 122
Jerk blends, 111
joint support, 88–91
juniper, 26, 30

K

kani pepper (*Xylopia aethiopica*), 42
kidney function, 27, 98–99
kidney tonics, **106–107**
Koleosho, Funke, 42, *42*

L

Latin America, 111
laurel family (*Lauraceae*), 15
lavender (*Lavandula angustifolia*)
    Cognitive Blend, 136–137
    medicinal uses of, **80–81**
    overview of, *38*, 64, *65*
leaves, 8, 10
Lemonade, Hot Ginger, 152
lignans, 20

M

mace (*Myristica fragrans*), 79

malotira (*Sideritis syriaca*), 142–143
masticha (*Pistacia lentiscus*), 143
measurements, 114, **114**
Medicinal Miso Soup, 147
medicinal uses
    blending for, 110–111
    for calm and focus, 92–94
    of curries, 150
    for digestion, 95–97
    disease prevention, 23–26
    drug interactions and, 26–27
    for heart health, 100–103
    for immune protection and defense, 84–87
    for kidney health, 27, 98–99
    overview of, **80–81**, 83, **106–107**
    for respiratory health, 103–105
    for skin, bones, and joints, 88–91
Mediterranean diet, 20, *21*
Mediterranean region, 6, **112**
memory, 94, **106–107**
Mexican oregano (*Lippia graveolens*)
    Not Necessarily Spicy Chili Blend, 140–141
Middle East, 7, **112**
milk, 144, 150
Mindful Pesto, 148
mint (*Mentha* spp.)
    Cognitive Blend, 136–137
    digestion and, 96–97
    medicinal uses of, **80–81**
    Mint and Chile Blend, 128–129
    Minty Yogurt Spread, 129
    overview of, *38*, 66, *66*, 67
    respiratory health and, 103–104
mint family (*Lamiaceae*), 14, 15, 142–143.
    See also holy basil
Miso Soup, Medicinal, 147
molasses, 123
mole blends, 111
molecular structure, 29, *29*
mung dal
    Sandeep's Kitchari, 151
mustard (*Brassica nigra*)
    Garlic Spread, 146
    Heart Healthy Blend, 134–135
    immune protection and defense and, 87
    Medicinal Miso Soup, 147

TAKE CARE NATURALLY
WITH MORE BOOKS FROM STOREY

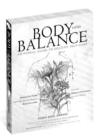

Body into Balance
by Maria Noël Groves

Achieve optimal health by learning to use herbs most effectively. Step-by-step photographs and in-depth instructions help you read the clues to your body's imbalances while teaching you how to minimize use of pharmaceuticals.

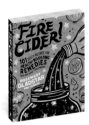

Fire Cider!
by Rosemary Gladstar

Spice up your healthcare regimen with this traditional immune-boosting elixir of apple cider vinegar and warming herbs. More than 70 herbalists share their favorite fire cider formulations and creative ways to get your daily dose.

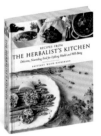

Recipes from the Herbalist's Kitchen
by Brittany Wood Nickerson

Generous proportions of familiar culinary herbs star in these scrumptious recipes for snacks, entrées, drinks, and desserts that are specially designed to meet the body's needs for comfort, nourishment, energy, and support through seasonal changes.

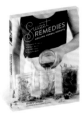

Sweet Remedies
by Dawn Combs

Make medicine that's a treat to take! Capture the health-boosting synergy of raw honey and medicinal herbs with recipes for safe, effective electuaries, oxymels, and infused honeys that address wellness needs, from heart health to cold and flu relief.

Join the conversation. Share your experience with this book, learn more about Storey Publishing's authors, and read original essays and book excerpts at storey.com. Look for our books wherever quality books are sold or call 800-441-5700.

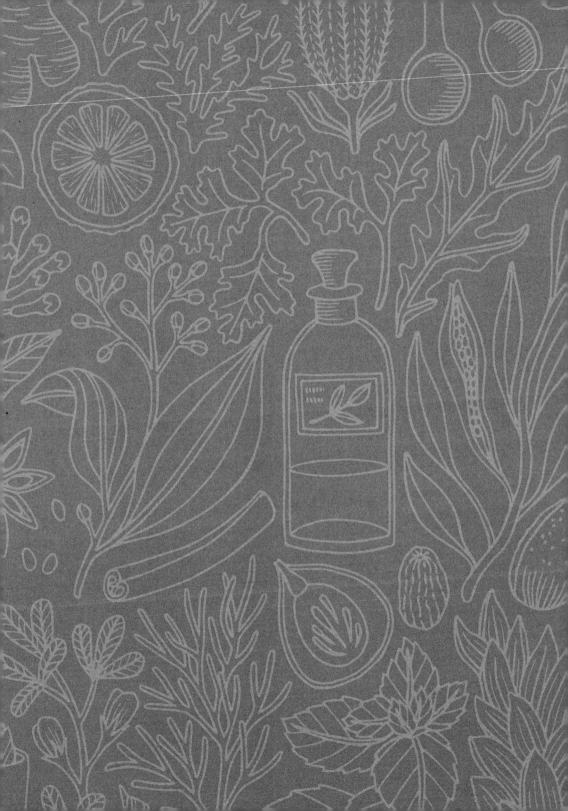